HIV

What Do I Do Now?: Infectious Diseases

SERIES EDITOR-IN-CHIEF

Mark S. Dworkin, MD, MPH & TM
Professor, Division of Epidemiology and Biostatistics
University of Illinois at Chicago
Chicago, IL, USA

FORTHCOMING VOLUMES IN THE SERIES
General Infectious Diseases

HIV

Edited by

Gregory D. Huhn
Associate Professor of Medicine, Rush University Medical Center;
Attending Physician, Division of Infectious Diseases, Cook County
Health, Chicago, IL, USA

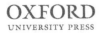

OXFORD
UNIVERSITY PRESS

OXFORD
UNIVERSITY PRESS

Oxford University Press is a department of the University of Oxford. It furthers
the University's objective of excellence in research, scholarship, and education
by publishing worldwide. Oxford is a registered trade mark of Oxford University
Press in the UK and certain other countries.

Published in the United States of America by Oxford University Press
198 Madison Avenue, New York, NY 10016, United States of America.

Library of Congress Cataloging-in-Publication Data
Names: Huhn, Gregory D., editor.
Title: HIV / [edited by] Gregory D. Huhn.
Other titles: HIV (Huhn) | What do I do now?
Description: New York, NY : Oxford University Press, [2021] |
Series: What Do I Do Now?: infectious diseases | Includes bibliographical references and index.
Identifiers: LCCN 2020031185 (print) | LCCN 2020031186 (ebook) |
ISBN 9780190088316 (paperback) | ISBN 9780190088330 (epub) |
ISBN 9780190088347 (online)
Subjects: MESH: HIV Infections—therapy | HIV Infections—complications |
Antiretroviral Therapy, Highly Active | Drug Resistance, Viral—drug
effects | Post-Exposure Prophylaxis—methods | Case Reports
Classification: LCC RA643.8 (print) | LCC RA643.8 (ebook) | NLM WC 503.2 |
DDC 614.5/99392—dc23
LC record available at https://lccn.loc.gov/2020031185
LC ebook record available at https://lccn.loc.gov/2020031186

DOI: 10.1093/med/9780190088316.001.0001

9 8 7 6 5 4 3 2 1
Printed by Marquis, Canada

Contents

Preface

As a third-year medical student rotating at Charity Hospital in New Orleans, I admitted a gentleman who appeared in his mid-50s, though his birthdate listed him in his late 30s. He said he was from New York; he could not actually tell us why he had come down to Louisiana, the burden of homelessness we suspected. He had been losing weight, swallowing food had been difficult for about a month, and his exam revealed obvious thrush. One of my first questions, do you have HIV? He told me no. I asked if he had ever been tested. Again, no. Our screening ELISA came back the next day, positive for HIV. We gave him the news, and he then told us that a doctor in New York diagnosed him with HIV several years ago, but he didn't believe it. He confided he had been traveling to several cities seeking repeat testing, hoping with each one he would finally hear the words, it's negative. This was early in 1995, just about 6 months before the breakthrough of combination antiretroviral therapy, a landmark year with the promise of health and a real future for many our patients. But at this moment, my patient simply asked me, "What do I do now?" My answer was of reassurance that we could treat his oral (and probable esophageal) candidiasis, but disappointingly I could not faithfully assuage his true plea, am I going to be alright.

We're taught early in our training to listen to our patients, and through this attentiveness often the path to diagnosis and hopefully healing will reveal itself. So 25 years later, now with the proven power of antiretroviral therapy (ART) to extend life span, as well as HIV prevention to turn back the threat of transmission, the compendium here flips this question, "What do I do now?" toward ourselves in examining a wide range of clinical, pharmacologic, mental health, behavioral, and social factors that impact contemporary care of persons living with HIV (PLWH). We have curated 29 case-based discussions from real patient encounters to take us as providers through the steps in first listening to the patient, then drawing on knowledge to date from clinical studies, guidelines, and expert experience to apply best practices and take home messages in shepherding our patients to greater health and equanimity.

This book is not intended to replace an HIV textbook or online manual, but rather complement it. I envision the vignettes and narratives in this book as a guidepost more toward thinking slow rather than fast. For most of us, we consider ourselves rational, analytical human beings. Yet, as exquisitely outlined by Daniel Kahneman and Amos Tversky, two psychologists lauded in behavioral economics (with a nifty Nobel Prize in Economics for Dr. Kahneman) who defined our internal mechanisms of decision-making, we actually spend almost all of our daily lives hovering in the thinking fast lane, deploying heuristics that fuel our intuitive reactions. By thinking slow, we engage reflection, problem-solving, and critical analysis in our decision-making process. As that medical student my fast thinking clicked in, I saw the thrush, treated it without hesitation, and essentially stopped digging literally and figuratively for more textured layers of my patient's immunological and environmental condition. But his plight stuck with me, and in this era we have the tools; let's start with readily available HIV RNA viral loads and integrative multidisciplinary case management models, respectively, to more deeply explore effective therapeutics, as well as wrap-around social services to stabilize mental health and hopefully reverse stigma. So I encourage readers to veer to the slow side of the shoulder in reading through these chapters, position yourselves as the patient's provider for the stories they tell, and appreciate the dissection, unraveling, and eventual hopeful restorative journey the authors achieve in encapsulating clarity and expert guidance toward these clinical challenges among our patients living today with HIV.

Contributors

Oluwatoyin M. Adeyemi, MD
Division of Infectious Diseases
Cook County Health
Rush University Medical Center
Chicago, IL, USA

Mariam Aziz, MD
Division of Infectious Diseases
Rush University Medical Center
Chicago, IL, USA

David E. Barker, MD, MPH
Division of Infectious Diseases
Department of Health Information
Systems
Cook County Health
Chicago, IL, USA

Robert K. Bolan, MD
Los Angeles LGBT Center
Los Angeles, CA, USA

Hillary Dunlevy, MD, MPH
Department of Medicine
Division of Infectious Diseases
University of Colorado Denver
Aurora, CO, USA

Rick Elion, MD
Department of Medicine
George Washington University
School of Medicine
Washington, DC, USA

Matthew J. Feinstein, MD, MSc
Division of Cardiology
Department of Medicine
Division of Epidemiology
Department of Preventive
Medicine
Northwestern University Feinberg
School of Medicine
Chicago, IL, USA

**L. Beth Gadkowski, MD,
MPH, MS**
Southeast AIDS Education and
Training Center
Division of Infectious Diseases and
Global Medicine
University of Florida
Gainesville, FL, USA

Estefania Gauto-Mariotti, MD
Department of Medicine
Cook County Health
Chicago, IL, USA

Ronnie M. Gravett, MD
Division of Infectious Diseases
University of Alabama at
Birmingham
Birmingham, AL, USA

Giorgos Hadjivassiliou, MD
Neighborhood Health Clinic
Alexandria, VA, USA

Connie Haley, MD, MPH
Southeast National
Tuberculosis Center
Division of Infectious Diseases and
Global Medicine
University of Florida
Gainesville, FL, USA

Patricia Heaslip, PA-C
Division of Infectious Diseases
Cook County Health
Chicago, IL, USA

Timothy J. Henrich, MD
Division of Experimental Medicine
Department of Medicine
University of California, San
Francisco Medical Center
San Francisco, CA, USA

Sybil Hosek, PhD
Department of Psychiatry
Division of Infectious Disease
Cook County Health
Chicago, IL, USA

Gregory D. Huhn, MD, MPHTM
Division of Infectious Diseases
Cook County Health
Rush University Medical Center
Chicago, IL, USA

Mamta K. Jain, MD, MPH
Division of Infectious Diseases and
Geographic Medicine
UT Southwestern Medical Center
Dallas, TX, USA

**Thana Khawcharoenporn,
MD, MSc**
Division of Infectious Diseases
Department of Internal Medicine
Faculty of Medicine
Thammasat University
Pathumthani, Thailand

Raphael J. Landovitz, MD, MSc
Division of Infectious Diseases
University of California Los
Angeles
Los Angeles, CA, USA

Ronald Lubelchek, MD
Division of Infectious Diseases
Cook County Health
Chicago, IL, USA

Jeanne Marrazzo, MD, MPH
University of Alabama at
Birmingham
Birmingham, AL, USA

Blake Max, PharmD
Ruth M. Rothstein CORE Center
University of Illinois at Chicago
College of Pharmacy
Chicago, IL, USA

**Jessica A. Meisner, MD,
MS, MSHP**
Division of Infectious Diseases and
Geographic Medicine
UT Southwestern Medical Center
Dallas, TX, USA

Monica Merçon, MD, MPH, PhD
Division of Infectious Diseases
Cook County Health
Chicago, IL, USA

Anna B. Moukouri Kouoh, CRNP
Department of Psychiatry and Behavioral Sciences
Johns Hopkins AIDS Psychiatry Service
Johns Hopkins Hospital
Baltimore, MD, USA

Khalil Nasser, MD
Midway Specialty Care Center Inc.
Fort Pierce, FL, USA

Juliana Netto, MD, MSc, PhD
LapClin/AIDS
National Institute of Infectious Diseases
Fundação Oswaldo Cruz—FIOCRUZ
Rio de Janeiro, Brazil

Gretchen Snoeyenbos Newman, MD
Division of Allergy and Infectious Diseases
Department of Medicine
University of Washington
Seattle, WA, USA

Arvind Nishtala, MD, MPH
Division of Cardiology
Department of Medicine
Northwestern University Feinberg School of Medicine
Chicago, IL, USA

Edgar T. Overton, MD
Division of Infectious Diseases
University of Alabama School of Medicine
Birmingham, AL, USA

Michael J. Peluso, MD
Division of HIV, Infectious Diseases, and Global Medicine
Department of Medicine
University of California, San Francisco Medical Center
San Francisco, CA, USA

Christian B. Ramers, MD, MPH
UC San Diego School of Medicine
Population Health
Family Health Centers of San Diego
San Diego, CA, USA

Moti Ramgopal, MD
Midway Specialty Care Center Inc.
Fort Pierce, FL, USA

Sarah A. Rojas, MD
Population Health
Family Health Centers of San Diego
San Diego, CA, USA

Paul G. Rubinstein, MD
Section of Hematology Oncology
Department of Medicine
Cook County Health
Rush University Medical Center
Chicago, IL, USA

Huma Saeed, MBBS
Division of Infectious Diseases
Rush University Medical Center
Chicago, IL, USA

Carlos A. Q. Santos, MD, MPHS
Division of Infectious Diseases
Rush University Medical Center
Chicago, IL, USA

Nicholas P. Schweizer, EdD, LCADC, LCPC
Departments of Psychiatry and
Behavioral Services and Internal
Medicine
Johns Hopkins AIDS Psychiatry
Service
Johns Hopkins Hospital
Baltimore, MD, USA

Beverly E. Sha, MD
Division of Infectious Diseases
Rush University Medical Center
Chicago, IL, USA

Rebekah Shephard, APRN
Department of Psychiatry
Ruth M. Rothstein CORE Center
Cook County Health
Chicago, IL, USA

Glenn Treisman, MD, PhD
Department of Psychiatry and
Behavioral Sciences
Department of Internal
Medicine
Johns Hopkins Hospital
Baltimore, MD, USA

Antonio E. Urbina, MD
Department of Medicine
Icahn School of Medicine
Mount Sinai Hospital
New York, NY, USA

Pamela Vergara-Rodriguez, MD
Psychiatry and Internal
Medicine
Ruth M. Rothstein CORE
Center
Cook County Health
Chicago, IL, USA

Brian R. Wood, MD
Division of Allergy and Infectious
Diseases and
Department of Medicine
University of Washington
Seattle, WA, USA

Fariba Younai, DDS
Section of Oral Medicine and
Orofacial Pain
UCLA School of Dentistry
Los Angeles, CA, USA

1 "The condom broke and I'm tired of worrying about HIV"

Sybil Hosek and Raphael J. Landovitz

Warren, a 22-year-old, gay-identified, cisgender male, presents at your walk-in sexual health clinic. He reports that he had a sexual encounter the day before and the condom broke during receptive anal intercourse. Warren reports that this was a new male sexual partner, and that he is unaware of the partner's HIV status. The patient reports that he isn't frequently sexually active but does have occasional "hookups" once or twice per month. Review of the medical record is significant for past history of rectal gonorrhea last year and pharyngeal chlamydia at age 20. Warren expresses concern that he may have been exposed to HIV this time and also reports that he is "tired of worrying about HIV every time that I want to have sex."

What Do You Do Now?

This patient has presented with a possible HIV exposure that needs to be evaluated with a thorough history of the sexual event in order to ascertain the level of HIV risk posed. Warren reports that the sexual encounter involved condomless insertive oral intercourse and receptive anal intercourse. A condom was used at the onset of the anal intercourse but broke at some point prior to ejaculation. The event occurred approximately 24 hours ago while Warren was visiting friends in a nearby city. Upon arriving home, he immediately presented to the clinic. Warren does not know the HIV status of the sexual partner and does not have any mechanism to contact him. Given the type of sexual activity and the inability to establish whether the sexual partner is living with HIV, the exposure should be considered of substantial risk of transmitting HIV; Warren should be evaluated for nonoccupational postexposure prophylaxis (nPEP).

Nonoccupational postexposure prophylaxis involves the use of antiretroviral medications for HIV-uninfected people with an exposure to blood, genital secretions, or other body fluid that may potentially contain HIV outside of the occupational setting (i.e., not a needle-stick in a hospital). While no randomized, placebo-controlled trials of nPEP have been conducted for reasons of feasibility and ethics, data from animal models, mother-to-infant transmission trials, observational studies of healthcare exposures, and case reports of nPEP use support recommendations that nPEP initiated within 72 hours after exposure and continued for 28 days reduces the risk of acquiring HIV. A systematic review and meta-analysis of 25 nonhuman primate studies found the risk of seroconversion was lowered by 89% among animals exposed to postexposure prophylaxis (PEP) compared with those who did not receive it.

For Warren, who is still within the exposure window of less than 72 hours, it is important to rule out preexisting HIV infection. A history and physical examination to evaluate for any clinical signs and symptoms of acute HIV infection should be performed. For expediency, a rapid HIV antibody or combined antigen/antibody (Ag/Ab) blood test should be conducted in the clinic. In addition, a laboratory-based Ag/Ab test could be completed along with an HIV RNA test if locally available. However, in cases where rapid results are not available or feasible, nPEP should be provided immediately even in the absence of HIV test results. In fact, because

HIV infection can occur very quickly, providers may prefer to provide the first dose of PEP at the clinic while they complete their initial evaluation.

In 2016, the US Centers for Disease Control and Prevention (CDC) updated the guidelines for nPEP to include preferred as well as alternative 3-drug antiretroviral medication regimens for otherwise healthy adults and adolescents (Table 1.1). Rather than providing a "starter pack" and requiring patients to schedule a subsequent appointment, clinicians are encouraged to provide the full 28-day course of PEP to decrease patient burden. Studies suggested that acceptance of PEP and completion rates are better among those given the full course compared to those given starter packs and asked to follow up subsequently with another or a different provider visit. The ultimate goal is to prescribe nPEP in a manner that is urgent, recognizes that exposure to HIV is a medical emergency, and gets the first dose of antiretroviral agent into the patient as soon as possible.

If the exposure source is actually known to be a person living with HIV (PLWH), the provider should attempt to interview that person or obtain that source person's medical records with consent to determine the history of antiretroviral therapy (ART) use and most recent viral load. This information can guide the choice of initial nPEP or modifying nPEP ART in response to resistance testing results if a viremic source PLWH agrees to further evaluation to account for potentially resistant virus.

In addition to HIV testing and nPEP prescription, testing for rectal, urethral, and pharyngeal bacterial sexually transmitted infections (STIs), syphilis, as well as hepatitis A, B, and C should be completed. For cisgender women, urine and cervical swabs for STIs should be collected along with

TABLE 1.1   **Preferred and Alternative nPEP Regimens**

Preferred Regimen	Alternative Regimen
Tenofovir disoproxil fumarate (TDF) (300 mg) with emtricitabine (FTC) (200 mg) once daily *PLUS* Raltegravir (RAL) (400 mg) twice daily *OR* dolutegravir (DTG) (50 mg) daily	Tenofovir disoproxil fumarate (TDF) (300 mg) with emtricitabine (FTC) (200 mg) once daily *PLUS* Darunavir (DRV) (800 mg) *AND* ritonavir (RTV) (100 mg) once daily

a pregnancy test for those of childbearing potential. Patients who are not already immune to hepatitis A and B should be vaccinated.

Warren's laboratory-based HIV and STI tests are still pending, but the rapid test completed in the clinic comes back negative. Warren is counseled about the initial test results and common side effects associated with the drugs. Given the importance of daily adherence for 28 days, additional adherence support strategies should be considered, including pillboxes, cell phone alarms/reminders, and follow-up text messages or phone calls based on patient preference. Pending test results will be shared with Warren as they come in, and a follow-up appointment is scheduled in approximately 3 weeks to discuss future prevention options. Warren fills his prescription on site, takes his first dose in the clinic, and leaves with the remainder of the medication in hand.

WHAT ARE THE NEXT STEPS IN THIS CASE?

Warren returns for his follow-up appointment 25 days after his first dose of nPEP was provided in the clinic. He reports experiencing mild gastro-intestinal symptoms during the first week of taking the medication, but that these subsequently resolved. Warren mentions that he did travel out of town the previous weekend and forgot to bring his pill bottle with him, thus missing two doses. At this point, it would be appropriate to take a complete sexual history from Warren if it was not obtained at the initial emergency visit and continue discussions around HIV prevention strategies that may work best for Warren, including HIV preexposure prophylaxis (PrEP).

The US Food and Drug Administration (FDA) approved the use of once daily tenofovir and emtricitabine (TDF/FTC; Truvada˚) as oral PrEP for HIV prevention in adults in 2012 based on the results from several efficacy trials. Open-label effectiveness studies have since supported that TDF/FTC reduces the risk of HIV by over 95% when taken consistently. On May 15, 2018, the US FDA expanded the indication to include adolescents weighing at least 35 kg who are at risk for HIV infection based on data from the Adolescent Trials Network (ATN) 113 study. In addition to clinical recommendations by the CDC and World Health Organization (WHO), the US Preventive Services Task Force (USPSTF) recently released an "A" rating for PrEP among adolescents and adults who are at high risk of HIV acquisition.

In October 2019, a new regimen of once daily tenofovir alafenamide with emtricitabine (TAF/FTC; Descovy') was also approved for HIV prevention among those at risk for HIV through anal sex, but not approved for vaginal sex. In the DISCOVER trial, a Phase 3 randomized trial comparing TDF/FTC to TAF/FTC, TAF/FTC was found to be noninferior (i.e., as effective) to TDF/FTC in preventing HIV among cisgender men who have sex with men (MSM) and transgender women. However, several researchers and public health officials have recently called for TDF/FTC to remain the first-line formulation for daily oral PrEP in all populations at risk of HIV exposure.

In addition to a once daily regimen, "on-demand" or "event-driven" TDF/FTC has been shown to be effective. In the IPERGAY study, taking 2 pills prior to sex and 2 single doses 24 and 48 hours after sex ("on-demand dosing" or "2-1-1") was shown to be highly effective (86%) among MSM. Subsequent open label trials also supported the efficacy of on-demand PrEP, with no reported HIV infections in either the daily or on-demand arm of the ANRS PREVINIR study. In July 2019, the WHO updated its PrEP guidance to include the use of event-driven PrEP by MSM. However, once daily oral dosing remains the only regimen currently approved by the US FDA.

Warren is excited about the possibility of transitioning from nPEP to PrEP. Warren describes the frequency of his sexual activity (1 or 2 times per month) as well as the fact that he only missed a couple of doses of his daily PEP regimen. Based on this, Warren would like to try daily PrEP. The goal for Warren is to seamlessly transition him from PEP to PrEP. He has 3 more doses of nPEP to complete. During today's visit, HIV antibody testing should be completed, and, if feasible, an HIV RNA test may be helpful in ensuring that Warren has not acquired HIV infection during the course of nPEP.

Warren's previous laboratory results are reviewed, and he is already immune to hepatitis A and B and does not have hepatitis C. Baseline PEP laboratory values demonstrated a negative rapid plasmin reagin (RPR) test and no evidence of gonorrhea or chlamydia in his pharynx, rectum, or urethra. Warren is advised that while he is taking PrEP, he will be tested for HIV and bacterial STIs quarterly regardless of symptoms, and his kidney function will be monitored every 6–12 months. He will be required to come in for his testing/blood work before refilling his prescription every 3 months. He likes the idea of more consistent sexual healthcare. It is important to discuss with Warren instructions for missed doses, including that he should take the dose "late" as long as it is the same calendar day that it was due; otherwise, he should skip that dose and resume regular dosing the following day. It is also important to convey to Warren that there is some forgiveness to missed dosing without significant loss of protection as long as an average of 4 or more doses weekly are ingested. Warren is reminded that PrEP does not protect him against bacterial STIs, so condoms are still recommended for all genital contact to protect against those infections. During future visits, Warren's sexual activity and HIV transmission risk should continue to be evaluated with an open discussion of discontinuing PrEP or moving to an on-demand regimen, depending on his current situation. These discussions should also serve to remind Warren that if he does decide to stop PrEP, then subsequently wants to start again, HIV testing must be conducted prior to restarting.

KEY POINTS TO REMEMBER

- Potential exposures to HIV should be considered as emergencies and PEP provided urgently.
- There is no need to wait for initial HIV testing results before dispensing PEP because a 3-drug regimen is being used.
- There is no need to have a "break" between PEP and PrEP, particularly if HIV transmission risk is ongoing.
- No more than 3 months of TDF/FTC PrEP should be prescribed at a time, with required interval testing for HIV, STIs, and other safety parameters before represcribing.
- TAF/FTC may be appropriate for PrEP for those with preexisting kidney or bone disease or those at high risk for such complications.

Further Reading

Baeten JM, Donnell D, Ndase P, et al. Antiretroviral prophylaxis for HIV prevention in heterosexual men and women. *N Engl J Med*. 2012 Aug 2;367(5):399–410.

Centers for Disease Control and Prevention. Updated guidelines for antiretroviral postexposure prophylaxis after sexual, injection drug use, or other nonoccupational exposure to HIV—United States, 2016. *Ann Emerg Med*. 2016 Sep 1;68(3):335–338.

Centers for Disease Control and Prevention: US Public Health Service: Preexposure prophylaxis for the prevention of HIV infection in the United States—2017 Update: a clinical practice guideline. https://www.cdc.gov/hiv/pdf/risk/prep/cdc-hiv-prep-guidelines-2017.pdf. Published March 2018.

Grant RM, Lama JR, Anderson PL, et al. Preexposure chemoprophylaxis for HIV prevention in men who have sex with men. *N Engl J Med*. 2010 Dec 30;363(27):2587–2599.

Hosek SG, Landovitz RJ, Kapogiannis B, et al. Safety and feasibility of antiretroviral preexposure prophylaxis for adolescent men who have sex with men aged 15 to 17 years in the United States. *JAMA Pediatr*. 2017 Nov 1;171(11):1063–1071.

Irvine C, Egan KJ, Shubber Z, Van Rompay KK, Beanland RL, Ford N. Efficacy of HIV postexposure prophylaxis: systematic review and meta-analysis of nonhuman primate studies. *Clin Infect Dis*. 2015 Jun 1;60(suppl 3):S165–S169.

Jain S, Krakower DS, Mayer KH. The transition from postexposure prophylaxis to preexposure prophylaxis: an emerging opportunity for biobehavioral HIV prevention. *Clin Infect Dis*. 2015 Jun 1;60(suppl 3):S200–S204.

Krakower DS, Daskalakis DC, Feinberg J, Marcus JL. Tenofovir alafenamide for HIV preexposure prophylaxis: what can we DISCOVER about its true value? *Ann Intern Med*. 2020 Jan 14;172(4):281–282.

Molina JM, Capitant C, Spire B, et al. On-demand preexposure prophylaxis in men at high risk for HIV-1 infection. *N Engl J Med*. 2015 Dec 3;373(23):2237–2246.

Thigpen MC, Kebaabetswe PM, Paxton LA, et al. Antiretroviral preexposure prophylaxis for heterosexual HIV transmission in Botswana. *N Engl J Med*. 2012 Aug 2;367(5):423–434.

2 "I just found out that I have HIV"

Ronald Lubelchek

A 26-year-old male with 2 days of fever and chest rash walks into the Sexually Transmitted Infection (STI) clinic. His sexual history is notable for having 6 male partners with whom he has had unprotected receptive anal sex over the last 2 months. His temperature is 38.8°C, heart rate is 110 beats per minute, and blood pressure is 105/70 mm Hg. Pertinent positive examination findings include injected sclera and an erythematous, nonpruritic exanthem on his chest and back, with few lesions on his soles. You send urine, throat, and rectal samples for gonorrhea/chlamydia nucleic acid testing, a syphilis enzyme immunoassay, and viral hepatitis serologies. As you consider the differential, a staff person knocks on the door to inform you that the patient's point-of-care HIV test is reactive. You plan to send supplemental testing to confirm the HIV diagnosis and treat for secondary syphilis. Should you start him on antiretroviral therapy (ART) today or simply refer him to an HIV clinic for further evaluation?

What Do You Do Now?

Use of ART to treat HIV leads to extensive benefits at both the individual and the public health levels. By gaining a more complete appreciation of the many benefits of ART, clinicians can make informed decisions regarding when to initiate ART for patients recently diagnosed with HIV. This chapter reviews both the immunologic and longevity gains attributable to ART, as well as ART's effectiveness for preventing onward HIV transmission. Considering its effectiveness and due to improvements in ART's potency, along with concomitant declines in ART-related adverse effects and pill burden, the pendulum of when to initiate ART has swung toward early initiation. Same day-of-diagnosis ART initiation, or rapid start within several days of diagnosis, has moved from the realm of research to clinical care. In the United States, the Centers for Disease Control and Prevention (CDC) estimated that only 53% of persons living with HIV (PLWH) have achieved virologic suppression. In recognition of the need to improve HIV-related outcomes, the US government has launched its Ending the HIV Epidemic (EtHE) initiative, which seeks a 90% reduction in the number of annual new HIV diagnoses by 2030. HIV treatment, inclusive of a rapid start of ART, represents one of the EtHE initiative's fundamental pillars. This chapter reviews the benefits of ART, highlights data supporting same-day/rapid ART initiation and discuss its real-world application.

THE INDISPUTABLE BENEFITS OF ART

Prior to the development of effective therapy, HIV infection led to progressive depletion of CD4 T lymphocytes and a resultant severe and often fatal immune compromise. Virologic suppression achieved via use of ART allows for CD4 count increases and immunologic recovery. Crucially, baseline/nadir CD4, to some extent, mediates the degree of CD4 rebound. The HIV Outpatient Study (HOPS) investigators, for example, demonstrated that having a CD4 value greater than 200 cells/mL^3 at baseline strongly correlated with achieving a CD4 value greater than 750, roughly in the middle of the normal range, during subsequent follow-up.

Just as ART allows for immunologic recovery, numerous longitudinal cohort studies have documented ART-related declines in mortality and associated improvements in longevity for PLWH. HOPS investigators demonstrated that mortality rates for their cohort members declined from 29/100 person-years of follow-up in 1995, to 9/100 person-years in 1997, a change largely attributable to the availability of multidrug combination ART regimens. Over time, as ART has improved, PLWH have continued to enjoy further reductions in mortality. The North American AIDS Cohort Collaboration on Research and Design demonstrated that the life expectancy for PLWH at age 20 increased from 36 to 51 years from 2000–2002 to 2006–2007.

Improvements in access to and efficacy of ART have also provided a critical tool for preventing onward HIV transmission. From longitudinal cohort study to randomized controlled trial, the notion that viral suppression represents a robust means of preventing HIV transmission has been repeatedly confirmed. The PARTNER study followed nearly 800 sero-discordant men who have sex with men (MSM) couples, of whom the PLWH couple member was on suppressive ART with a most recent HIV viral load less than 200 copies/mL. Over nearly 1600 couple-years of observation, inclusive of couples engaging in more than 76,000 episodes of condom-less anal sex, investigators identified zero linked transmissions of HIV to seronegative partners.

HOW EARLY IS EARLY ENOUGH?

The dramatic individual, as well as public health, benefits associated with ART have begged the question of how early is early enough with respect to ART initiation (Figure 2.1). To answer this question, the Strategic Timing of Antiretroviral Treatment (START) trial during 2009 to 2013 enrolled 4685 ART-naïve PLWH, with a median CD4 of 651 cells/mL[3] at study

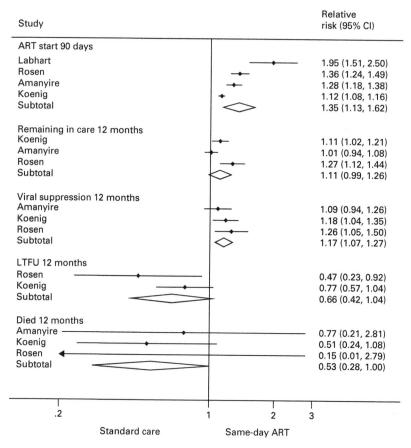

FIGURE 2.1 Outcomes from randomized trials comparing same-day ART start versus standard of care. ART, antiretroviral therapy; CI, confidence interval; LFTU, Lost to follow up. Reprinted with permission of Wolters Kluwer Health Incorporated from Ford N, Migone C, Calmy A, et al. Benefits and risks of rapid initiation of antiretroviral therapy. *AIDS (London, England).* 2018;32(1):17–23.

entry. Study staff randomized patients to early (CD4 > 500) versus deferred ART (CD4 < 350 cells/mL³). Early versus deferred ART patients reached the study's primary composite endpoint of serious AIDS or non–AIDS-related event and/or death, at an event rate of 0.6 versus 1.4 per 100 person-years (hazard ratio 0.43, 95% CI 0.30 to 0.62, p < .0001). The START study and the similar TEMPRANO study have definitively demonstrated the benefit of early ART initiation, even for relatively immunologically intact patients.

WHAT IS RAPID START AND WHICH DATA SUPPORT ITS USE?

Per the World Health Organization (WHO) guidelines on rapid initiation of ART, rapid ART start comes in two varieties: same-day initiation of ART or near-immediate initiation, within a week of a patient's HIV diagnosis. While the START and similar TEMPRANO studies demonstrated the benefit of starting ART in patients with relatively preserved CD4 counts, additional studies have assessed the benefit of same-day or rapid initiation of ART for recently diagnosed PLWH. Spurred by concern over the possibility that patients may fail to return for care between HIV testing and ART initiation visits, the Rapid Initiation of Antiretroviral Therapy (RapIT) study, conducted in South Africa during 2013 to 2014, randomized newly diagnosed HIV patients to initiation of treatment at their first HIV clinic visit versus standard of care, which entailed additional clinic visits over 2 to 4 weeks for completion of various pretreatment assessments. Investigators considered the proportion of patients who achieved an undetectable HIV viral load at 10 months as the study's primary endpoint, while also assessing various secondary endpoints, including the proportion on ART in less than 90 days from randomization. Of the 377 enrolled patients, 64% versus 51% of patients randomized to the same-day versus the standard ART initiation achieved viral suppression (HIV RNA < 400 copies/mL) at 10 months (relative risk [RR] 1.26, 95% CI 1.05–1.50); additionally, 81% versus 64% (RR 1.27, 95% CI 1.12–1.44) had started on ART by 90 days and remained in care at 10 months in the 2 groups, respectively.

A similar same-day ART initiation study conducted in Haiti during 2013 to 2015 revealed comparable outcomes. The Groupe Haitian d'Etude du Sarcoma da Kaposi at des Infections Opportunistas (GHESKIO)clinic in Haiti randomized newly diagnosed PLWH with CD4 counts less than

500 cells/mL^3 to either same-day ART or standard therapy. Patients in this study were screened for tuberculosis (TB) with a chest x-ray and needed to pass a simple 7-question ART readiness survey. Fifty-three versus 44% in the same-day versus standard ART groups reached the primary endpoint of retention in care and maintenance of virologic suppression (HIV RNA < 50 copies/mL) at 12 months (adjusted RR for reaching endpoint of 1.24, 95% CI 1.06–1.41, p = .008); further, significantly more patients in the standard treatment arm versus the same-day start arm died (5.6% vs. 2.9%, RR 0.43, 95% CI 0.19–0.94, p = .033).

Observational studies conducted in more resource-replete settings have corroborated findings of the RapIT and Haiti rapid ART initiation studies. At the San Francisco General Ward 86 Clinic, investigators compared newly diagnosed HIV patients referred to their Rapid ART Program Initiative for HIV Diagnoses (RAPID) program within less than 30 days from diagnosis versus patients with more delayed referral to their rapid ART initiation program. The clinic team provided patients with adherence training, benefits counseling, near-term clinic follow-up, reminder phone calls, and an ART starter pack. Investigators found that patients enrolled in the RAPID program soon after diagnosis versus those with delayed referral to the program achieved virologic suppression in 65 versus 170 days from diagnosis (p < .001). Importantly, this study did not select only "ideal" patients to target for same-day ART; more than 50% of patients reported substance abuse, 48% had major mental health diagnoses, and 31% reported unstable housing.

In addition to the apparent clinical benefits, including improved rates of ART initiation, virologic suppression, and care retention, rapid ART initiation confers benefits for patients with acute HIV infection. Starting acutely infected patients on treatment leads to a reduction in the size of the reservoir of latently infected memory CD4 T cells, which correlates with a reduction in the viral plasma RNA set point, as well as lower levels of immune activation. These findings underscore the particular benefit that immediate ART may have in the setting of acute/early HIV infection.

PRACTICAL CONSIDERATIONS FOR SAME-DAY/RAPID ART

All same-day/rapid ART initiation programs reported in the medical literature incorporated an assessment of a newly diagnosed PLWH with readiness to start ART. Treatment interruptions, even when planned, have been shown to worsen clinical outcomes, which underscores the importance of integrating an assessment of readiness into same-day/rapid ART initiation efforts.

Utilization of a team-based patient care approach also represents a crucial best practice for same-day/rapid ART programs. While sites implementing same-day ART often cannot provide all pertinent wraparound services during a first visit, most ensure that patients have timely access to comprehensive behavioral health services, along with health education and benefits counseling. Further, many such programs assign patients a navigator who can direct patients as they become acquainted with the many challenges of the medical care delivery system. Given typical restrictions to specialty service access, it is relevant that some programs have made use of primary care providers operating with structured algorithmic support, along with near-term HIV specialist follow-up.

Lack of access to comprehensive laboratory results prior to ART initiation also represents a common reality in the same-day/rapid start arena. Rapid ART start prescribers will often lack CD4, HIV viral load, HLA B5701, HIV genotype, and even renal function results as they devise a treatment plan. While lack of baseline HIV genotype results raises the theoretical concern that pretreatment drug resistance (PDR) may reduce treatment response, the overall efficacy of rapid initiation strategies largely invalidates this concern. While rates of PDR have increased globally, the majority of PDR mutations confer non-nucleoside reverse transcriptase inhibitor (NNRTI) resistance, and most nation-specific guidelines have shifted away from NNRTI-containing first-line ART regimens. Improved virologic outcomes seen in rapid/same-day start patients in resource-limited settings, despite lack of routine access to HIV genotype data, underscores the countervailing benefit that early initiation of therapy likely has, even in the context of possible NNRTI PDR.

In more resource-replete settings, first-line ART for treatment-naïve PLWH has largely shifted toward regimens employing a nucleos(t)ide reverse transcriptase inhibitor (NRTI) backbone plus integrase inhibitor (InI). In settings that use NRTI plus InI first-line ART, PDR has not been shown to detrimentally effect same-day ART initiation outcomes. The New Orleans–based Crescent Care Start Initiation team found that 23% of their rapid start patients did have PDR, of which 86% conferred NNRTI resistance. For the study's 2 patients whose virus did harbor baseline M184V lamivudine (3TC)/emtricitabine (FTC) resistance-conferring mutations, both achieved virologic suppression. Due to concern for PDR, most guidelines recommend use of an ART regimen inclusive of a nucleos(t)ide backbone plus either an InI or boosted darunavir for same-day/rapid ART initiation. The DIAMOND study evaluated the utility of using a boosted protease-inhibitor based regimen in the setting of rapid ART initiation. This single-arm study enrolled 109 recently diagnosed PLWH to begin a single-tablet regimen comprised of tenofovir alafenamide (TAF)/FTC/darunavir/ cobicistat within 14 days of diagnosis. Investigators reported that 84% in the intention-to-treat analysis and 96% of observed patients maintained virologic suppression (HIV RNA < 50 copies/mL) at 48 weeks. Table 2.1 provides a summary of key same-day/rapid ART–related guidelines.

TABLE 2.1 **Same-Day/Rapid Antiretroviral Therapy (ART) Guidelines Review**

Agency	Month/ Year Issued	Same-Day/Rapid ART Recommended (Yes/No/ Other)	Preferred Same-Day/Rapid Start ART Regimen(s)
World Health Organization	July 2017	Yes/patients with advanced disease (CD4 < 200 cells/ mL^3) to be prioritized	Per country-specific guidelines
US Department of Health and Human Services	July 2019	Guidelines describe same-day/rapid ART initiation as investigational	Boosted darunavir, or DTG, plus tenofovir and FTC or 3TC
International AIDS Society	July 2018	Yes, but with reservations	Boosted darunavir or DTG or bictegravir plus tenofovir and FTC or 3TC
European AIDS Clinical Society	November 2019	ART for all PLWH; same-day start to be considered on case-by-case basis	Non–NNRTI-based regimen

Abbreviations: DTG, dolutegravir; FTC, emtricitabine; 3TC, lamivudine.

CAVEATS TO CONSIDER

Providers should consider several key caveats when contemplating same-day/rapid ART initiation. Due to concerns about TB and/or cryptococcosis-related immune reconstitution inflammatory syndrome (IRIS), providers should screen patients—particularly those living in or having immigrated from an area of higher endemicity—for these opportunistic infections (OIs). In the South African RapIT study, providers screened patients for TB via a symptom questionnaire and, if needed, same-day chest radiography and rapid expectorated sputum evaluation, with TB patients withdrawn from the study. Cryptococcal disease was similarly screened for in both the RapIT and Haiti/GHESKIO clinic rapid ART initiation studies. While TB and possible central nervous system OIs should exclude patients from same-day ART consideration, other OIs should not be considered contraindications for rapid ART initiation. The AIDS Clinical Trials Group 5164 study found that patients with OIs, excluding TB, had reduced mortality when starting ART within 2 weeks of initiating OI treatment.

Other key considerations in choosing a same-day ART regimen include the presence of possible chronic kidney disease (CKD); chronic, active Hepatitis B; and/or pregnancy. In resource-replete settings, CKD poses less of a concern given that ART regimens with TAF-based nucleoside backbones have approval by the Food and Drug Administration for patients with creatinine clearances greater than 30 mL/min. In rapid ART start studies set in resource-limited settings that employ tenofovir disoproxil fumarate–based ART, patients with CrCl less than 50 mL/min were safely changed to either zidovudine or abacavir-based therapy if HLA-B5701 negative. Due to the need to treat co-occurring hepatitis B infection, if present, without changing therapy, ART regimens that contain TDF or TAF plus FTC/3TC may be preferred for use in the same-day/rapid ART initiation context. Additionally, for pregnant women living with HIV, providers should refer to specific pregnancy-related HIV treatment guidelines, and prior to same-day/rapid ART initiation providers should obtain point-of-care pregnancy testing on patients with childbearing potential.

CONCLUSION

Research has demonstrated the clinical efficacy of same-day/rapid ART initiation for treatment-naïve PLWH. While starting ART prior to availability of baseline resistance test data may seem counterintuitive, use of potent first-line regimens with a high barrier to resistance largely neutralizes this concern. Prescribers considering same-day/rapid ART initiation need to assess patient readiness for therapy, as well as integrate the patient's care with comprehensive wraparound services. Used in this context, same-day/rapid ART initiation represents a powerful tool to improve outcomes for PLWH.

KEY POINTS TO REMEMBER

- Same-day/rapid start of ART can improve rates of ART initiation, virologic suppression, and care retention.
- Baseline resistance as not been shown to worsen outcomes when starting same day ART.
- Readiness to start treatment should be assessed prior to same-day ART initiation.
- Same-day ART should be provided in the context of full complement of wraparound services

---

Further Reading

Ford N, Migone C, Calmy A, et al. Benefits and risks of rapid initiation of antiretroviral therapy. *AIDS (London, England)*. 2018;32(1):17–23.

Halperin J, Butler I, Conner K, et al. Linkage and antiretroviral therapy within 72 hours at a federally qualified health center in New Orleans. *AIDS Patient Care STDs*. 2018;32(2):39–41.

Huhn GD, Crofoot G, Ramgopal M, et al. Darunavir/cobicistat/emtricitabine/tenofovir alafenamide in a rapid initiation model of care for HIV-1 infection: primary analysis of the DIAMOND study. *Clin Infect Dis*. 2019 Dec 27; pii:ciz1213. doi:10.1093/cid/ciz1213. [Epub ahead of print]

Koenig SP, Drovil N, Dévieux JG, et al. Same-day HIV testing with initiation of antiretroviral therapy versus standard care for persons living with HIV: a randomized unblinded trial. *PLoS Med*. 2017; e1002357.

Pilcher CD, Ospina-Norvell C, Dasgupta A, et al. The effect of same-day observed initiation of antiretroviral therapy on HIV viral load and treatment outcomes in a US public health setting. *J Acquir Immune Defic Syndr.* 2017;74(1):44–51.

Rosen S, Maskew M, Fox MP, et al. Initiating antiretroviral therapy for HIV at a patient's first clinic visit: the RapIT randomized controlled trial. *PLoS Med.* 2016;13(5):e1002015.

World Health Organization. *Guidelines for Managing Advanced HIV Disease and Rapid Initiation of Antiretroviral Therapy.* Vol. 2019. Geneva, Switzerland: World Health Organization; 2017.

3 "I hear there is a new medicine that means I don't need to take so many pills?"

Gretchen Snoeyenbos Newman and Brian R. Wood

A 55-year-old cisgender man was diagnosed with HIV in 2005 and started a regimen of efavirenz/emtricitabine (FTC)/tenofovir disoproxil fumarate (TDF) in 2006. He missed doses due to depression and experienced virologic failure. Genotypic resistance testing detected new M184V and K103N substitutions. He switched to ritonavir-boosted atazanavir with FTC/TDF and experienced jaundice, which prompted a change to ritonavir-boosted darunavir plus FTC/TDF (a regiment of 3 pills per day) in 2009. He reports excellent adherence since that time. His HIV RNA (viral load) has remained suppressed on this regimen, and his current CD4 count is 560 cells/mm^3. He is a current tobacco smoker and has hypertension treated with a thiazide diuretic, hyperlipidemia treated with low-dose rosuvastatin, and lumbar radiculopathy, for which he is considering an epidural steroid injection. He asks, "Can I take fewer medicines?"

What Do You Do Now?

OPTIMIZING TREATMENT FOR HIV

Improved antiretroviral therapy (ART) has allowed the majority of persons with HIV (PWH) who engage in care and adhere to treatment to expect a near-normal life span. This success means that many PWH will take ART for 30 to 40 years or more and will experience the challenges of modern aging, including medical comorbidities, polypharmacy, and treatment fatigue. Clinical care for HIV now predominantly focuses on helping navigate these challenges and optimizing ART regimens to minimize toxicity and maximize quality of life.

For PWH with routinely suppressed viral loads, we define a successful ART switch as one in which the viral load remains suppressed and other factors improve, such as pill burden, ease of regimen, short-term side effects, long-term toxicity risk, or drug-drug interactions. Other indications for a regimen switch may include pregnancy or plans to conceive, insurance coverage changes, or new or worsening medical comorbidities such as renal insufficiency.

In the case presented, the impetus for an ART switch stems from a patient-directed desire for treatment simplification plus a provider-motivated goal to decrease potential drug-drug interactions, especially between ritonavir and a corticosteroid injection, improve serum lipids, and reduce cardiovascular risk.

HOW NECESSARY OR URGENT IS AN ART SWITCH?

Providers generally base the necessity or urgency of an ART switch on the severity of potential toxicities of the current regimen components. In general, older antiretrovirals (ARVs) with higher risks of long-term side effects take highest priority for a switch. For example, a person taking an older nucleoside reverse transcriptase inhibitor (NRTI) (i.e., zidovudine or stavudine) or older protease inhibitor (PI) (e.g., lopinavir, saquinavir, nelfinavir, fosamprenavir, or indinavir) should always switch to newer, less-toxic agents. A rare exception is a patient with extensive drug resistance and no effective alternatives to zidovudine based on the resistance profile.

Switching from other agents may be less urgent, but merits consideration. For example, guidelines in the United States no longer recommend efavirenz, nevirapine, cobicistat-boosted elvitegravir, atazanavir, or boosted darunavir as first-line agents for ART-naïve PWH. For individuals taking one of these ARVs, we generally perform a detailed review for side effects, which may be subtle, and drug-drug interactions, including over-the-counter medications. We then discuss potential benefits versus risks of a switch to newer options. If a person reports tolerating one of these ARVs and the viral load remains suppressed, then a change is not required, but we have a low threshold to recommend a switch if foreseeable benefits exist.

One example of potential advantages of an ARV update is efavirenz. This non-nucleoside reverse transcriptase inhibitor (NNRTI) can cause subtle or overt central nervous system or mental health side effects, including suicidality, and may also raise lipid levels and reduce vitamin D levels. Many, though not all, individuals feel better after a switch to a different agent, even when no overt side effects are reported. Thereby, we often encourage a switch from efavirenz to a newer NNRTI or to an integrase strand transfer inhibitor (INSTI). Similarly, replacing a boosted PI with an alternate ARV often reduces gastrointestinal side effects, drug-drug interactions, and metabolic side effects. Here, we favor a switch to dolutegravir or bictegravir, particularly if there may be underlying NRTI resistance or if the ARV or resistance history is unknown.

This is a critical point: Regimens anchored by a boosted PI, as the patient in the case is taking, require a thorough preswitch assessment because these drugs have a relatively high barrier to resistance, and a switch to a regimen with relatively lower barrier to resistance, such as raltegravir, elvitegravir, or an NNRTI, may raise the risk of virologic failure. A similar caution is advised if considering a change from bictegravir or dolutegravir, which have relatively high barrier to resistance, to an ARV with a relatively lower barrier. In these situations, we switch to an agent of equivalent barrier to resistance or ensure a patient has no history of NRTI or other resistance that may compromise the new regimen before making a switch (discussed more in best practices for a switch).

Another common clinical question is which patients should switch from TDF to tenofovir alafenamide (TAF). Due to reduced plasma levels of circulating metabolites as compared to TDF, TAF likely induces lower risk of renal proximal tubulopathy and decreased adverse effects on bone mineral density. For persons with risk factors for TDF-induced renal insufficiency, the change from TDF to TAF becomes more pressing, and we typically recommend an update. For other individuals, we have a low threshold to recommend a switch, but see less urgency.

For the patient in the case, switching to a regimen that avoids TDF and a pharmacokinetic booster would be ideal, but a thorough review of all past resistance testing should occur first.

CHANGING FROM A 3-DRUG REGIMEN TO A 2-DRUG REGIMEN

Classically, ART regimens have included 3 active agents in order to maintain a suppressed viral load and prevent the development of resistance. Recently, the US Food and Drug Administration (FDA) approved 2 dual ART formulations: dolutegravir/rilpivirine and dolutegravir/lamivudine. Studies of both of these dual-ARV options as maintenance ART for carefully selected individuals with virologic suppression demonstrated noninferiority as compared to traditional 3-drug ART regimens. Providers should recommend these options only for individuals with durable viral suppression (at least 6 to 12 months), no resistance to either of the drugs in the new combination, and no hepatitis B co-infection.

BEST PRACTICES FOR A SAFE SWITCH

The most important step prior to any switch is to compile a complete ART history, including every prior regimen and the reason for stopping or switching, particularly eliciting any drug intolerances and virologic failures, as well as a review of all past resistance test results. All results must be reviewed—not simply the most recent—because mutations detected years ago may be archived in proviral DNA, and these remain clinically relevant even if not detected on more recent testing.

Not infrequently, a person's ART history or the results of prior resistance tests are unavailable, yet the patient and/or the provider wish to make a switch to ART. Persons who have taken only 1 or 2 prior regimens, who are confident they have not experienced prior virologic failures, and who have excellent adherence can generally switch ART without issue. For PWH with possible past virologic failures and resistance yet no available records, a new regimen ought to contain the same number of active agents and equivalent barrier to resistance as the currently effective regimen, though pill burden can sometimes be improved through changes to combination pills. Again, individuals taking dolutegravir, bictegravir, or a boosted PI should not switch to a regimen of relatively lower barrier to resistance if there is concern for or documented NRTI resistance. When prior resistance testing is unavailable, a DNA genotype can be obtained even when the HIV RNA is undetectable, but a composite of past RNA genotype results is preferred as DNA genotypes have lower sensitivity and specificity.

Clinicians often grapple with what to recommend for a patient with an isolated M184V or M184I NRTI mutation, as raised in the case in this chapter. Based on personal experience and the DAWNING study, we feel comfortable simplifying a patient's regimen to dolutegravir or bictegravir plus FTC/TAF if M184V/I is the only NRTI mutation and if the patient has recent suppressed or relatively low viral loads (below 100,000 copies/mL). If the viral load is detectable above 100,000 copies/mL, some clinicians, including us, add an additional ARV agent (NNRTI or boosted PI), then drop this additional agent once the viral load becomes undetectable.

Other key factors to consider when selecting a new ART regimen include drug-drug interactions, food requirements, potential for pregnancy, pill burden, and insurance coverage. Before a switch from tenofovir (TAF or TDF) to an alternative agent, co-infection with hepatitis B must be ruled out to ensure that co-infected patients receive treatment that is adequate for both HIV and hepatitis B.

Following any ART change, an HIV RNA level should be drawn after 4 weeks to confirm continued suppression. A phone call to the patient a few days after the switch allows the provider to address unanticipated logistical complications or side effects. Finally, developing a contingency plan in case the new medication is not available or not tolerated prevents lapses in adherence.

WHAT SHOULD WE DO FOR OUR PATIENT?

The patient in our case wishes to simplify his regimen and reduce pill burden. His comorbidities affect ART selection, including risk factors for cardiovascular events and renal disease. We would avoid regimens containing abacavir because it may raise cardiovascular risk and because it is less active than TDF or TAF with the M184V mutation, and we would avoid TDF to reduce renal risk. Furthermore, we would eliminate a pharmacokinetic booster to avert serious interactions with the corticosteroid injection and interactions with the statin, which may allow more options to treat hyperlipidemia. Recent data suggest that treatment with bictegravir or dolutegravir with TAF may lead to more weight gain as compared to treatment with other agents; however, the mechanism and clinical implications require future study. If switching to bictegravir, dolutegravir, and/or TAF, we would emphasize counseling about lifestyle modifications to reduce this risk.

Given the patient's desire for "fewer medicines," we would prioritize selection of a 1-pill, once-per-day regimen. Bictegravir/FTC/TAF would be an optimal choice and, as described in this chapter, would likely maintain viral suppression in the setting of the M184V mutation, particularly in someone with durable viral suppression and excellent adherence. If access to bictegravir/FTC/TAF were an issue, dolutegravir plus FTC/TAF would be an effective alternative. We would counsel the patient regarding lifestyle modifications to reduce the risk of weight gain with either of these regimens.

If considering dual-ART maintenance therapy, we would not consider dolutegravir/lamivudine due to the M184V mutation. Dolutegravir/rilpivirine could be considered if there were no other drug-drug interactions and if the food requirement were not an issue.

KEY POINTS TO REMEMBER

- The goal of an ART regimen change is typically to improve quality of life or reduce short- or long-term medical risks while maintaining virologic suppression.
- Prior to an ART regimen switch, it is imperative to review a number of clinical factors, including the individual's history of prior ART regimens and tolerability, all prior resistance test results, full medication list for potential drug-drug interactions, medical comorbidities and hepatitis B status, as well as food requirements, pregnancy or pregnancy potential, and insurance coverage.
- When switching from a regimen of relatively high barrier to resistance (e.g., a combination anchored by bictegravir,

dolutegravir, or a boosted PI) to a regimen of relatively lower barrier to resistance (e.g., one with a first-generation NNRTI, elvitegravir, or raltegravir as the anchor), it is especially important to confirm past resistance and virologic failure history to verify that the NRTI backbone remains active.

- If switching from a standard 3-drug ART regimen to a 2-drug maintenance combination, it is crucial to make sure the 2 drugs in the new regimen are fully active, and we make sure one of the agents in the new regimen has a relatively high barrier to resistance.

- Prior to making an ART regimen switch, we counsel the patient about potential risks, the possibility of switching back to their prior regimen if they do not tolerate the new one, and a follow-up plan that includes a phone call or visit to ensure the switch is made correctly and a repeat viral load after approximately 4 weeks.

Further Reading

Aboud M, Kaplan R, Lombaard J, et al. Dolutegravir versus ritonavir-boosted lopinavir both with dual nucleoside reverse transcriptase inhibitor therapy in adults with HIV-1 infection in whom first-line therapy has failed (DAWNING): an open-label, non-inferiority, phase 3b trial. Lancet Infect Dis. 2019;19(3):253–264.

Eron JJ, Young B, Cooper DA, et al. Switch to a raltegravir-based regimen versus continuation of a lopinavir-ritonavir-based regimen in stable HIV-infected patients with suppressed viraemia (SWITCHMRK 1 and 2): two multicentre, double-blind, randomised controlled trials. Lancet. 2010;375(9712):396–407.

Llibre JM, Hung CC, Brinson C, et al. Efficacy, safety, and tolerability of dolutegravir-rilpivirine for the maintenance of virological suppression in adults with HIV-1: phase 3, randomised, non-inferiority SWORD-1 and SWORD-2 studies. Lancet. 2018;391(10123):839–849.

van Wyk J, Ajana F, Bisshop F, et al. Switching to DTG+3TC fixed dose combination (FDC) is non-inferior to continuing a TAF-based regimen (TBR) in maintaining virologic suppression through 24 weeks (TANGO Study). Presented at the Tenth IAS Conference on HIV Science; July 20–24, 2019; Mexico City, Mexico.

Wood BR. Switching antiretroviral therapy in the setting of virologic suppression: a why and how-to guide. Infect Dis Clin North Am. 2019;33(3):693–705.

4 "I'm not that good with taking pills every day"

Blake Max

A 44-year-old man living with HIV is seen for an initial appointment after relocating due to job transfer. The patient was diagnosed in 2005, and his current antiretroviral regimen is darunavir 600 mg twice daily plus ritonavir 100 mg twice daily plus rilpivirine 25 mg daily and dolutegravir 50 mg twice daily. He reports taking this regimen for the past few years, has no complaints, and has had no recent hospitalizations. He states excellent adherence, which is confirmed by pharmacy refill records, although he admits to occasionally missing the evening dose of the twice-daily medications. His only medications are antiretrovirals, which he takes with food. He does not take any over-the-counter medications and does not complain of any side effects. Routine laboratory tests are ordered; the results all are within normal range except the HIV viral load at 3517 copies/mL.

What Do You Do Now?

EVALUATION AND MANAGEMENT OF
MULTIDRUG-RESISTANT HIV

The goal for antiretroviral treatment–experienced patients is the same for treatment-naïve patients: to achieve an undetectable viral load. Ideally, this can be achieved by selecting at least 2, but preferably 3, fully active drugs for the treatment-experienced patient. The selection of active drugs should be based on both past and present drug resistance tests and previous antiretroviral drug history. However, selecting active drugs can be challenging in patients who have been prescribed multiple regimens and have a history of virologic failure. There are over 40 individual or combination antiretroviral agents available that target HIV reverse transcriptase, protease, integrase, or viral entry. Regardless of drug or drug class, HIV has the ability to develop drug resistance and often cross resistance within a drug class. For developed countries, virologic failure has become increasingly less common due to more potent, better tolerated, and higher barrier to resistance HIV treatment regimens. However, there are still many patients living with HIV who entered care when treatment was not as effective, drugs were not as tolerable, and drug resistance was more common than it is today. The medication history reveals the patient has been prescribed multiple antiretroviral regimens in the past and has had multiple HIV drug resistance test.

Past medical records are obtained, baseline HIV genotype was wild type (no drug-resistant mutations) at the time of HIV diagnosis. His HIV viral load was 78,000 copies/mL, CD4+ T-lymphocyte count was 350 cells/mL; all other laboratory values were within normal limits, and he was initiated on tenofovir disoproxil 300 mg/emtricitabine 200 mg/efavirinez 600 mg (Atripla®) once daily. His clinical course remained stable over the next 5 years, HIV viral load remained undetectable, and CD4+ T-lymphocyte count plateaued at 740 cells/mL. In 2010, his HIV viral load was detectable (1567 copies/mL and 3421 copies/mL) after 2 successive clinic visits 4 weeks apart. An HIV genotype test was ordered, and M184V and K103N mutations in HIV reverse transcriptase were detected. The interpretation of the genotype is high-level resistance to lamivudine and emtricitabine (nucleoside reverse transciptase inhibitors, NRTIs) and efavirenz and nevirapine (non-nucleoside reverse transcriptase inhibitors, NNRTIs). The patient admitted to poor adherence due to loss of insurance and inability to pay for medications. Based on results/interpretation of the genotype, the primary care provider initiated tenofovir disoproxil 300 mg/emtricitabine 200 mg (Truvada*, an NRTI) once daily plus lopinavir/ritonavir 200 mg/50 mg (Kaletra*, a protease inhibitor [PI]) 2 tablets twice daily plus raltegravir 400 mg twice daily (Isentress*, an integrase strand transfer inhibitor [INSTI]). The new regimen contained 3 active antiretrovirals, and the patient was enrolled for the state AIDS drug assistance program.

The patient responded well to the salvage regimen; however, after 6 years, he developed persistent low-level viremia (viral load fluctuated between 500 and 2500 copies over 10 months). At each clinic visit during this time of viremia, the patient admitted difficulty taking medications twice daily and agreed to improve adherence after each clinic encounter. Another HIV genotype with HIV integrase was ordered after failing to achieve undetectable HIV viral load. The results from the genotype showed reverse transcriptase mutations K65R, M184V; protease enzyme mutations K20M, M36I, V82A, L90M; and integrase mutation N155H. The interpretation of the genotype (including mutations from previous genotype) was high-level resistance to all NRTIs except zidovudine, high-level resistance to efavirenz and nevirapine (NNRTIs), moderate-to high-level resistance to ritonavir-boosted atazanavir and lopinavir/ritonavir (PI), and high-level resistance to raltegravir and elvitegravir (INSTIs). Based on this information, the previous provider changed the regimen again to darunavir/ritonavir (PI) 600 mg/100 mg twice daily plus dolutegravir (INSTI) 50 mg twice daily plus rilpivirine (NNRTI) 25 mg daily, for a total of 3 active drugs.

Now that the treatment history and previous HIV resistance tests have been obtained, the patient should be educated on the importance of medication adherence, particularly the evening doses that are occasionally missed. A follow-up viral load check in 4 weeks is ordered. There are a number of factors that contribute to virologic failure, and they should be addressed before a regimen change occurs. Factors such as comorbid conditions (i.e., chemical dependency, mental health, neurocognitive disease); pill burden; adverse effects/toxicity; insurance coverage/drug cost; drug interactions; food requirements; patient understanding/interpretation of medication directions; and prescription errors are examples that can alter therapeutic drug levels or interfere with medication adherence, which is the primary reason for virologic failure. In some cases, there are no identifiable barriers, and the patient has excellent medication adherence but is still unable to reach the desired goal of undetectable viral load. The adherence assessment is performed, and no identifiable barriers were identified other than occasionally missing the evening dose of twice-daily medications; the follow-up HIV viral load was 2015 copies/mL.

There are 2 tests to determine antiretroviral drug resistance, and both require a plasma viral load of at least 500–1000 copies/mL. The clinician could order another HIV genotype with integrase and select a new antiretroviral regimen based on results from this test and previous tests. Another option is an HIV phenotype; however, this test is generally not preferred due to high cost, limited laboratories that can perform the test, and slower turnaround time. In certain clinical scenarios, HIV phenotype can be helpful for antiretroviral treatment-experienced patients (particularly patients with exposure to multiple regimens) and those who have a prior history of numerous drug-resistant mutations. Viral replication in different concentrations of drug are compared to a wild-type laboratory strain of HIV. Results are reported as a "fold change," which represents relative resistance to antiretroviral medications. The higher the fold change is, the greater the drug resistance will be. Drug susceptibilities are reported as sensitive, resistant, or resistance possible, which can guide the clinician in selecting active drugs. The advantage of HIV phenotype in this case is that the results may show some drugs that are sensitive that may have been overlooked or not expected to be active if a standard HIV genotype was performed.

The insurance for this patient would not cover an HIV phenotype. Therefore, the decision is to order another HIV genotype with integrase, and the results showed one new mutation (E138A) in the reverse transcriptase. This mutation is significant for high-level resistance to rilpivirine and low-level resistance to etravirine (both are NNRTIs). Given this information and results from previous genotypic tests, it is up to the clinician to construct a salvage regimen by determining if any active drugs are available. Some clinicians will consider continuing lamivudine or emtricitabine despite the presence of an M184V mutation (from historical genotype). In general, the development of drug resistance should be avoided; however, there are some immunological and clinical benefits associated with the M184V mutation. There are data to support the M184V mutation results in decreased viral fitness by reducing HIV reverse transcriptase processivity and hypersensitivity to other NRTIs, such as tenofovir and zidovudine. Because this mutation impairs viral replication and can increase susceptibility to other NRTIs, the thought is that once it is detected, it should remain. This can be achieved by prescribing either lamivudine or emtricitabine in the regimen.

The goal remains to identify at least 2 and preferably 3 active drugs from different classes of antiretrovirals for this patient. One class of antiretrovirals that the patient has not been exposed to are HIV entry inhibitors. This class has 3 drugs that are approved by the Food and Drug Administration (FDA) and another in late stages of clinical development. They do not appear to be antagonistic; therefore, co-administration of more than 1 can be used in the class. Enfuvirtide (Fuzeon®) was FDA approved in 2003 and must be reconstituted and administered subcutaneously (1 mL) twice daily. Injection site reactions and twice-daily administration are significant barriers to adherence. Enfuvirtide is a 35–amino acid synthetic protein that binds to HIV gp41 (HIV envelop protein) and inhibits fusion between virus and target cell membrane (CD4-T-lymphocyte). Maraviroc (Selzentry®) is a CCR5 co-receptor antagonist that inhibits viral entry. Maraviroc binds to C-C chemokine receptor type 5 (CCR5) coreceptor on the host cell surface, causing a conformational change and thus preventing HIV from binding to the co-receptor. Viral entry involves attachment to the CD4 host cell receptor, followed by interaction with another cell surface co-receptor (CCR5 or C-X-C chemokine receptor type 4 [CXCR4]). To determine which co-receptor the virus uses to gain cell entry, viral tropism must be determined. The test to determine viral tropism is called the HIV Trofile® test; at this time, only 1 laboratory in the United States can perform this test. The HIV Trofile test will determine if the virus is CCR5-tropic, in which case maraviroc would be active, or CXCR4-tropic or dual/mix-tropic (virus can use both co-receptors), in which case maraviroc would not be active. A Trofile test was ordered for this patient, and 1 month later the report came back dual/mix-tropic.

The third HIV entry inhibitor approved for HIV treatment is ibalizamab (Trogarzo®), which is an immunoglobulin (Ig) G monoclonal antibody that binds to domain 2 of the CD4-T-lymphocyte receptor. Binding of ibalizumab to the CD4+ receptor inhibits viral entry by steric hindrance but does not interfere with normal immune function. Ibalizumab is only available as an intravenous infusion and requires a loading dose of 2000 mg on day 1, followed by 800 mg IV infusion every 2 weeks. This medication not only requires a dedicated patient to make twice-monthly infusion appointments, but also dedicated clinical staff and site to administer and monitor this drug. Fostemsavir is an oral prodrug of temsavir, which binds directly to the viral envelop gp120 protein and blocks the first step of entry, which is viral attachment to the host CD4+ T-lymphocyte receptor. Fostemsavir is not FDA approved but is in the late clinical stages of development as a 600-mg, twice-daily oral tablet that has minimal drug interactions and appears to be well tolerated.

After review of the patient's HIV genotypes and antiretroviral treatment history, the clinician is left with a few options to consider. Although the patient has not been exposed to any entry inhibitors, they do not appear to be good options at this time. Maraviroc would not be active due to dual/mix tropism, enfuvirtide is not optimal because of twice-daily injections, ibalizumab would be challenging because of bimonthly clinic visits to receive an intravenous infusion, and fostemsavir is not FDA approved at this time. However, there are some treatment options that can provide a desired 3 active drug regimen. The PI darunavir would be active based on no darunavir-associated mutations reported on any previous genotype. It has been shown in a clinical trial with boosted darunavir that patients exposed to PIs (our patient was exposed to lopinavir/ritonavir) who do not harbor any darunavir-associated mutations once-daily boosted darunavir is safe, effective, and tolerable. Although the patient has significant resistance to the NNRTI class (K103N, E138A), these mutations do not impact doravirine, a new NNRTI approved by the FDA in 2018. The patient has resistance to first-generation INSTI (raltegravir and elvitegravir) based on N155H mutation. A clinical trial has shown that dolutegravir 50 mg twice daily is active for patients with prior INSTI exposure, including patients with N155H mutation. Therefore, based on the patient's historical genotypes and drug history, a salvage regimen of doravirine 100 mg once daily plus boosted darunavir (darunavir 800 mg/cobicistat 150 mg [Prezcobix®]) once daily plus dolutegravir 50 mg twice daily should provide 3 active drugs. Fortunately, 2 of the 3 drugs are once daily, and the patient will need education with emphasis on the importance of taking dolutegravir twice daily. This regimen will consist of 4 tablets, thus minimizing pill burden.

Despite history of the M184V mutation, lamivudine and emtricitabine will not be continued due to patient preference for minimizing pill burden and the ability to construct a salvage regimen containing 3 active drugs. In this case, the clinician must weigh the clinical benefit of continuing selective drug pressure to maintain the M184V mutation versus adding an additional pill and drug cost to the regimen. If the patient is unable to tolerate one of the recommended antiretrovirals, Descovy* (tenofovir alafenamide [TAF] 25 mg/emtricitabine 200 mg) can be considered. Despite previous history of K65R mutation selected by tenofovir disoproxil, there is in vitro data to support TAF, a new tenofovir prodrug, that appears to have partial activity. Improved pharmacokinetic properties of TAF compared to tenofovir disoproxil allow for higher intracellular target cell drug concentrations, which might be able overcome resistance observed in patients with K65R mutation. The presence of the K65R mutation is associated with intermediate- to high-level resistance to all NRTIs except zidovudine and possibly TAF. Zidovudine, although it must be dosed twice daily and has significant short-term and long-term side effects, could also be considered an active drug for this patient if changes need to be made.

KEY POINTS TO REMEMBER

- Drug-resistant testing should be performed when the HIV viral load is greater than 500–1000 copies/mL and the patient is taking antiretroviral therapy.
- Knowledge of previous antiretroviral drug-resistant tests and past antiretroviral drug history is critical for constructing a new treatment regimen.
- Selection of an antiretroviral drug regimen for treatment-experienced patients requires at least 2, but preferably 3, active drugs, with the goal to achieve undetectable viral load.
- Adherence barriers must be assessed when patients are viremic on antiretroviral therapy.
- Consultation with an HIV expert is recommended when complex drug-resistant mutations are present.

Further Reading

Cahn P, Fourie J, Grinsztejn B, et al. Week 48 analysis of once-daily vs. twice-daily darunavir/ritonavir in treatment-experienced HIV-1-infected patients. *AIDS.* 2011;25(7):929–939.

Castagna A, Maggiolo F, Pence G, et al. Dolutegravir in antiretroviral-experienced patients with raltegravir- and/or elvitegravir-resistant HIV-1: 24-week results of the phase III VIKING-3 study. *J Infect Dis.* 2014;210(3):354–362.

Este JA, Telenti A. HIV entry inhibitors. *Lancet.* 2007;370 (July 7):81–88.

Miller V, Stark T, Loeliger AE, Lange JMA. The impact of the M184V substitution in HIV-1 reverse transcriptase on treatment response. *HIV Med.* 2002;3:135–145.

Panel on Antiretroviral Guidelines for Adults and Adolescents. Guidelines for the use of antiretroviral agents in adults and adolescents with HIV. Department of Health and Human Services. http://www.aidsinfo.nih.gov/ContentFiles/ AdultandAdolescentGL.pdf. Accessed December 11, 2019 .

Shafer RW, Schapiro J. HIV-1 drug resistance mutations: an updated framework for the second decade of HARRT. *AIDS Rev.* 2008;10(2):67–84.

Wensing AM, Calvez V, Ceccherini-Silberstein F, et al. 2019 update of the drug resistance mutations in HIV-1. *Top Antivir Med.* 2019;27(3):111–121.

5 A "false-positive" HIV test?

Michael J. Peluso and Timothy J. Henrich

A 45-year-old man presents for a new patient visit.
Eighteen months ago, he was informed that a male
sexual partner tested positive for syphilis, and he
was treated empirically as a contact a month later.
He did not follow up for his test results and moved
out of state soon after. Over the last year, he became
increasingly concerned about his HIV status, and this
led to him abstain from sexual activity. His examination
is unremarkable except for mildly enlarged cervical
lymph nodes. A fourth-generation HIV antigen/antibody
(Ag/Ab) test is positive, but a concurrent plasma HIV
RNA test result is "detected, less than 40 copies." With
the patient's permission, you learn from the health
department that 18 months prior, his test results
showed a positive fourth-generation Ag/Ab test with
a concurrent plasma HIV RNA of 18,000, and they had
tried unsuccessfully to contact him for several months.
A repeat plasma HIV RNA the next day is "target not
detected," and the CD4 count is 650. He denies ever
taking antiretroviral therapy (ART). He asks you whether
the prior testing represents "false positives" or whether
he has been cured of HIV.

What Do You Do Now?

HIV ELITE CONTROL

Individuals capable of naturally controlling HIV infection in the absence of ART represent both a diagnostic and a management challenge for the treating clinician. In this chapter, we review what is known about the epidemiology, biology, and clinical outcomes of individuals across the clinical spectrum of natural HIV control and provide suggestions for the management of such individuals in a clinical setting.

DEFINITION AND EPIDEMIOLOGY OF NATURAL CONTROL OF HIV INFECTION

A small percentage of persons living with HIV are able to maintain some level of virologic and immunologic control of HIV infection without ART, defined here as "natural control" of HIV infection. In general, these individuals demonstrate considerable variability in both the degree and the duration of control. The spectrum ranges from partial control, typically with plasma HIV RNA levels (i.e., viral loads) in the hundreds or thousands of copies per milliliter of plasma ("viremic" controllers), to those demonstrating stricter control of the virus, with plasma levels below the limit of detection on standard assays ("elite" controllers) (Figure 5.1). Some individuals maintain control for years or decades, while others spontaneously lose control and develop escalating plasma viremia. Similarly, some controllers will maintain immunologic function ("long-term nonprogressors") for a sustained duration, while others will exhibit CD4+ T-lymphocyte count decline despite maintenance of low or undetectable plasma HIV RNA levels without ART. As a result, the identification, monitoring, and management of natural HIV controllers is challenging.

HIV elite control is a rare phenomenon, with estimates suggesting that 1% or fewer people living with HIV will exhibit this phenotype. A larger proportion of individuals exhibit viremic than elite control. Both phenotypes were described prior to the availability of widespread, effective ART in individuals who were living with HIV but demonstrated low or unquantifiable levels of virus. Modern clinical HIV practice often involves frequent testing and early treatment with widely available ART, which has made it difficult to ascertain with certainty the modern epidemiologic

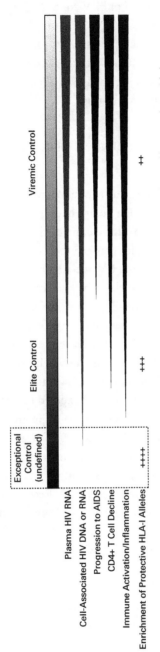

FIGURE 5.1 Schema showing the spectrum of natural HIV control and associated HIV burden, clinical progression, and immune characteristics.

trends and clinical progression of HIV control. Geographical trends of natural HIV control are also unclear. Many controllers were initially identified in the United States and Europe, but attempts to identify controllers in other settings have revealed unique challenges, such as undocumented or unreported ART use, that have made it difficult to determine the prevalence of this phenotype in such settings.

MECHANISMS AND DEVELOPMENT OF NATURAL HIV CONTROL

The exact mechanisms leading to natural control of HIV are not fully understood, but efforts over the last decade have provided insight into potential mechanisms through which natural control of HIV infection may be achieved and likely involves and interplay between the virus and host immune system. For example, natural control of HIV infection has been shown to be strongly associated with certain HLA alleles, which are considered "protective." These include HLA-B*27 and HLA-B*57 and perhaps HLA-B*58. While the mechanisms by which these alleles confer the ability to control HIV infection are likely to be multifactorial, in general they are thought to confer potent HIV-specific CD8+ T-cell activity that results in robust immune responses. These responses are typically polyfunctional, and lymphocytes exhibit relatively strong proliferative capacity when exposed to HIV antigen.

Much remains unknown about the development of elite control in the context of acute and early HIV infection. Controllers in several cohorts have demonstrated lower levels of plasma virus during early infection, suggesting the host immune responses during early infection are important in determining whether control is achieved. Recent work has described the acquisition of elite control in individuals diagnosed during early HIV infection; these individuals had protective HLA haplotypes but demonstrated variability in the peak viral load (~2000 to ~80,000 copies/mL) and the period of time over which they developed control (6 weeks to 6 months). Robust HIV-specific CD8+ T-cell responses appeared to play a role in each case, although no consistent patterns in these responses over time were present. Taken together, these studies suggest peak viremia may be lower in controllers, control may be achieved around the same time that noncontrollers reach the viral "set point," and a favorable host response, likely driven by CD8+ T cells, plays an important role in the attainment of the control.

CONSEQUENCES OF NATURAL HIV CONTROL AND POTENTIAL BENEFITS OF ART

Natural control of HIV infection is not without consequences. The association between untreated HIV infection and elevated levels of inflammation, microbial translocation, and immune dysfunction have been well described in noncontrollers. In general, these parameters improve with the administration of suppressive ART in noncontrollers. The Strategic Timing of Antiretroviral Treatment (START) and TEMPRANO studies showed that early initiation of ART is beneficial for individuals with HIV regardless of their CD4+ T-lymphocyte count.

Current guidelines strongly recommend ART initiation for controllers with declining CD4+ T-cell counts or evidence of HIV-related complications (https://aidsinfo.nih.gov/contentfiles/lvguidelines/AdultandAdolescentGL. pdf). However, there is substantial uncertainty regarding the appropriate management of elite controllers who have achieved and maintained undetectable viremia for a sustained duration of time. Over the last decade, it has become clear that many HIV controllers exhibit similar adverse consequences of HIV infection in the absence of ART. This includes persistent low-level viremia and signs of replication in the tissue, chronic inflammation, immune dysfunction, and non-AIDS diseases, including pulmonary and cardiovascular disease.

These findings have led to efforts to understand whether HIV controllers would benefit from the administration of ART. One observational study involved heterogeneous groups of controllers (some viremic, some aviremic) but demonstrated a clear signal toward a benefit of ART in terms of levels of viremia in plasma and gut tissue and markers of T-cell activation and dysfunction. Unfortunately, the START study was underpowered to study the impact of ART in controllers in a controlled fashion. For this reason, and in the era of efforts to "treat all" individuals living with HIV with ART, current practice in many settings is to offer ART to controllers even in settings in which they have demonstrated durable control and long-term nonprogression.

While the benefits of ART in noncontrollers are indisputable, the risk-benefit calculus remains somewhat unclear in the context of elite controllers. ART has become more tolerable over time, with a decreased pill burden and many fewer short-term side effects. However, there is growing evidence that even modern ART is not without risk. For example, tenofovir disoproxil fumarate, a commonly used nucleotide reverse transcriptase inhibitor (NRTI), is associated with cumulative renal and bone toxicity. Abacavir, another NRTI, and darunavir, a commonly prescribed protease inhibitor, have been associated with increased cardiovascular risk, although their precise relationship is controversial. Dolutegravir and bictegravir, second-generation integrase strand transfer inhibitors that have become a component of first-line regimens worldwide, and tenofovir alafanamide have recently been associated with weight gain in a subset of individuals. Moreover, it is generally accepted that individuals with undetectable plasma HIV RNA are unable to transmit HIV through sexual intercourse, although with the caveat that HIV persists in the semen of controllers. For these reasons, the risk-benefit calculus of treating all individuals exhibiting natural control of HIV infection remains complex, but many clinicians opt to initiate ART.

CLINICAL MANAGEMENT OF CONTROLLERS

Anticipation of future elite control in an individual with acute or early HIV infection is not currently possible, and therefore current guidelines strongly discourage delaying ART to see if a patient achieves spontaneous control.

However, scenarios in which individuals present with chronic undiagnosed HIV infection still occur. In such cases, the diagnosis of HIV infection should be confirmed with repeat fourth-generation Ab/Ag testing, and a current viral load should be obtained. While the case definition or elite control varies, most definitions at least require documentation of at least 3 plasma HIV RNA levels below the assay limit spanning at least a 1-year period. The clinician should assess whether the individual was ever exposed to ART, including whether they had previously taken HIV preexposure prophylaxis or postexposure prophylaxis. This should also include assessment of whether they have access to a partner's HIV medication. In some cases, the clinician might consider assessing ART drug levels to confirm that the individual is ART naïve.

We recommend that the clinician and patient participate in a discussion of the risks and benefits of ART initiation, including the risk of virologic progression or immunologic dysfunction in the absence of ART, risk of transmission to sexual partners if virologic progression occurs, as well as the potential risks of ART initiation. If the patient elects to defer ART, careful monitoring should occur with assessment of the plasma HIV RNA, CD4+ T-cell count, and surveillance for HIV-related complications every 3–6 months or with the development of new symptoms. Controllers initiating ART should be monitored according to the same guidelines as noncontrollers on ART. In cases in which an individual is confirmed to be ART naïve, has demonstrated sustained control of plasma HIV RNA, and has a robust CD4+ T-cell count, the clinician might consider referral to a research study.

"EXCEPTIONAL" ELITE CONTROL

Now that over 30 years have passed since the beginning of the HIV epidemic, it has led to questions about whether a more extreme phenotype of elite control should be further delineated. Recent work has identified a subset of elite controllers who are considered "exceptional" in that they have demonstrated decades of virologic control without immunologic decline. Descriptions of these rare individuals have provided insight into the most extreme phenotype of natural control. In general, these individuals exhibit very low or undetectable reservoirs (i.e., detectable HIV in peripheral blood cells or tissues that persists despite otherwise suppressive ART), low HIV-specific antibody responses, and low levels of T-cell activation. However, many questions remain. Because only a handful of exceptional controllers have been identified to date, it is unclear whether such individuals can maintain low levels of inflammation and immune dysregulation in the absence of ART, whether they exhibit ongoing activity or have spontaneously cleared tissue reservoirs of HIV infection, or whether they benefit from initiation of ART (or are harmed by withdrawal of ART). Even more importantly, questions remain about whether such individuals, although rare, may represent a true model of durable HIV control or, in some cases, functional cure of HIV infection.

- Natural control of HIV infection is a rare.
- Natural control of HIV infection represents a spectrum from those who exhibit exceptional control to those with ongoing viremia and clinical progression.
- Exceptional elite control of HIV infection may provide clues to how this unique phenotype may be recapitulated by HIV curative strategies.

Further Reading

Canoui E, Lecuroux C, Avettand-Fenoel V, et al. A subset of extreme human immunodeficiency virus (HIV) controllers is characterized by a small HIV blood reservoir and a weak T-cell activation level. *Open Forum Infect Dis.* 2017;4:ofx064.

Casado C, Galvez C, Pernas M, et al. Permanent control of HIV-1 pathogenesis in exceptional elite controllers: a model of spontaneous cure. *Sci Rep.* 2020;10:1902.

Gebara NY, El Kamari V, Rizk N. HIV-1 elite controllers: an immunovirological review and clinical perspectives. *J Virus Erad.* 2019 Sep 18;5(3):163–166.

Goulder P, Deeks SG. HIV control: is getting there the same as staying there? *PLoS Pathog.* 2018;14:e1007222.

Hatano H, Yukl SA, Ferre AL, et al. Prospective antiretroviral treatment of asymptomatic, HIV-1 infected controllers. *PLoS Pathog.* 2013;9:e1003691.

International HIV Controllers Study, Pereyra F, Jia X, McLaren PJ, et al. The major genetic determinants of HIV-1 control affect HLA class I peptide presentation. *Science.* 2010 Dec 10;330(6010):1551–1557.

Lopez-Galindez C, Pernas M, Casado C, et al. Elite controllers and lessons learned for HIV-1 cure. *Curr Opin Virol.* 2019 Oct;38:31–36.

Mendoza D, Johnson SA, Peterson BA, et al. Comprehensive analysis of unique cases with extraordinary control over HIV replication. *Blood.* 2012;119:4645–4655.

Morley D, Lambert JS, Hogan LE, et al. Rapid development of HIV elite control in a patient with acute infection. *BMC Infect Dis.* 2019;19:815.

Promer K, Karris MY. Current treatment options for HIV elite controllers: a review. *Curr Treat Options Infect Dis.* 2018 Jun;10(2):302–309.

6 "Do I need to use condoms if I'm taking my meds?"

Robert K. Bolan

John, age 35, comes in for his 6-month follow-up after starting antiretroviral treatment; his viral load testing was done 1 week ago. He has asked if his new partner, Jose, age 30, can be in the examination room for your meeting. John's initial CD4 count was 290; he started medication the day after his diagnosis and reports no missed doses. At 1 month, his viral load had sharply decreased, and by 3 months it was undetectable. You are happy to report that his 6-month viral load was also undetectable. Jose had been taking daily tenofovir/emtricitabine for about 1 year before he and John met. They are planning to be monogamous. John thinks that Jose needs to use preexposure prophylaxis (PrEP) indefinitely and still wants them to use condoms. Jose has heard about Undetectable = Untransmittable (U = U) and is overjoyed that John has a viral load that is undetectable. He wants to stop using PrEP.

What Do You Do Now?

THE HISTORY OF UNDETECTABLE
EQUALS UNTRANSMITTABLE

Until 1989 when Ho described a method for quantifying HIV-1 in the blood of infected persons, there was no direct way to measure the effectiveness of therapy. In addition, for roughly the first decade and a half of the epidemic, the drugs available could not durably suppress viral replication, so treatment as a means for ongoing prevention was not feasible. The first convincing evidence that treatment could reduce transmission came with the 1994 publication of the AIDS Clinical Trials Group (ACTG) 076 trial results. The study showed a 67.5% reduction in the risk of HIV maternal-infant transmission when mothers living with HIV were treated with zidovudine before and during labor and their newborns were treated with zidovudine for 6 weeks. However, it was already known that monotherapy with zidovudine eventually selected for resistance and led to treatment failure.

Musicco et al. reported that among their cohort of 436 HIV-seronegative women whose male partners living with HIV received zidovudine monotherapy as treatment, the rate of transmission to their female partners was lower only among those treated males who did not show signs of disease progression. Presumably, disease progression and HIV transmission were surrogates for treatment failure and viral rebound. Although this study provided further evidence that treatment could reduce transmission, it also showed that zidovudine monotherapy was not a long-term solution.

Studies with dual combinations of the few available single-class antiretroviral drugs were conducted, but it was not until 1995 when the first protease inhibitors were approved that things really began to change. Not only were these new drugs very potent antivirals, but also eventual failures of monotherapy suggested that combining drugs from different classes might further improve the efficacy and durability of treatment. In 1997, *Morbidity and Mortality Weekly Reports* reported the first decline in AIDS incidence, and this was attributed to these new treatment regimens.

In early 2008, the Swiss Commission on AIDS stated that, "The risk of sexual transmission of HIV is negligibly low if three conditions are met: (1) the HIV-infected patient is receiving antiretroviral therapy (ART) with excellent adherence; (2) blood viral load has consistently been undetectable

(<40 copies per mL) for more than 6 months; and (3) no STDs are present in either of the partners" (p. 165, https://translate.google.com/translate?hl=en&sl=fr&u=https://www.unige.ch/sciences-societe/socio/files/4814/0533/6055/Vernazza_2008.pdf&prev=search&pto=aue) The statement relied heavily on findings from the Rakai Project Study. Published in 2000, this study prospectively followed 415 heterosexual HIV-1–serodiscordant couples in rural Uganda for 30 months. Although there were 90 partners who seroconverted, none were among couples where the serum viral load of the partner living with HIV was less than 1500 copies/mL. There was a significant dose-response effect with respect to seroconversion, with 5.6% of the 90 seroconversions occurring when the viral load of the partner was between 400 and 3499 copies/ and increasing to 40% when the viral load was 10,000–49,000 copies/mL. The mere presence of a sexually transmitted infection did not significantly increase the rate of HIV transmission, but a history of genital discharge or dysuria in the partner living with HIV did, although this association did not remain significant in multivariable analysis.

At the XVII International AIDS Conference in Mexico City (July 2008), soon after the so-called Swiss statement was announced, Myron Cohen presented findings from the HIV Prevention Trials Network (HPTN) study 052, which further documented antiviral treatment as prevention. HPTN 052 enrolled 1763 serodiscordant, sexually active couples (98% were heterosexual) where CD4 count of the partner living with HIV was between 350 and 550 cells/mm³. They couples were randomized them to either begin ART immediately or delay ART until their CD4 count declined to 250 or less. At the time of its design, this study was one of many that sought to determine when the benefits of treatment outweighed the toxicity, tolerability, and adherence challenges of then-available treatment regimens. There was a 96.4% reduction in transmission in the early ART group compared to the delayed ART group. Importantly, this study characterized all seroconversions among the partners initially living without HIV to show whether they were phylogenetically linked to their partner living with HIV. Among the 46 linked infections documented in the study, 3 were in the early ART group and 43 were in the delayed ART group.

Building on this landmark work, the Partners Study enrolled 1166 serodiscordant couples in 14 European countries between September 2010 and May 2014. Of these, 888 couples (548 heterosexual and 340 men who have sex with men [MSM]) provided 1238 couple-years of follow-up. The aim of this study was to determine the risk of HIV transmission among serodiscordant couples who did not use condoms for penetrative anal or vaginal sex and where the viral load of the person living with HIV was less than 200 copies. There were no linked transmissions after 58,000 condomless sex acts. Overall, 94% of the eligible couple-years of follow-up were during periods when viral load measurements were less than 50 copies/mL; 6% were during periods when viral load measurement was between 50 and 200 copies/mL.

Due to a lower number of couple-years of on-study follow-up accrued for MSM compared to heterosexual couples, the investigators extended by 4 years the duration of follow-up for MSM. The extension study, called Partners2, enrolled an additional 630 MSM couples. Of all enrolled partners, 782 couples provided 1593 eligible couple-years of follow-up with a mean follow-up of 2.0 years. During this phase, 76,088 acts of anal sex were reported. Fifteen new HIV infections occurred among the partners not living with HIV, but none was phylogenetically linked to within-couple transmissions, resulting in a zero-transmission rate.

Finally, the Opposites Attract Study enrolled 343 serodiscordant MSM couples in Australia, Brazil, and Thailand. There were 16,800 condomless anal intercourse episodes reported with zero linked transmissions for 588.4 couple-years when the partner living with HIV had a plasma viral load of less than 200 copies/mL.

In 2016, the Prevention Access Campaign launched the message of U = U. The concept of U = U has become an axiom fully supported by scientific evidence that for individuals who are adherent to their ART regimens and whose viral loads are maintained at less than 200 copies/mL there is no sexual HIV transmission. Although controlled studies have not been done to establish an estimate of effectiveness, viral load suppression will also reduce transmission through needle sharing with injection drug use. The message of U = U is one of hope and removes stigma from living with HIV, provides further motivation to test, and, if positive, to initiate treatment and remain consistently adherent to it. The social, sexual, and re-productive lives of persons with HIV infection are transformed with the assured knowledge that they cannot transmit HIV. U = U should also prompt revision of existing statutes that allow HIV transmission prosecutions, especially where the accused person has a viral load that is undetectable. The promise of U = U removes one of the cruelest penalties HIV has exacted on the world in the last generation—stealing away the joy and affirmation of sexual intimacy.

THE DYNAMICS OF HIV REPLICATION: AN IMPORTANT VARIABLE

However, 2 things are still needed to convert the principle of U = U into pragmatic guidance for serodiscordant couples to prevent transmission. The first is to define what level of ART adherence is required for durable viral suppression. And the second is to establish the frequency of viral load testing to provide assurance that viral suppression is durable. The studies reviewed previously do not provide this guidance. Failure to adhere consistently to ART risks loss of viral control, and stopping ART leads to rapid viral rebound to levels where transmission can occur. As pointed out by Eisinger et al. in a recent *Journal of the American Medical Association* editorial, viral suppression at 6 months following initiation of ART is the shortest interval best supported by current evidence for predicting no transmission. Presumably, this time is required for removal of replication-competent virus from blood and genital compartments. Regardless of how long it takes, the fact that it is not immediate introduces the notion of "bridging PrEP" within a monogamous relationship to protect the uninfected partner until durable viral suppression has been achieved.

HIV replication and escape from viral suppression is a dynamic phenomenon wherein initial viral suppression and its maintenance are influenced by viral, medication, and adherence factors. Viral drug mutations, which can lead to incomplete or inconsistent suppression, may have been transmitted within the infecting founder virus species of a new infection and become archived by an initially suppressing ART regimen. Also, resistance mutations can develop over time with lapses in adherence or due to other factors that can affect drug absorption or metabolism. All such mutations may be further selected by minor lapses in adherence and lead to rising viral loads, which could differ among individuals. ART regimens vary in their mutation barriers, their metabolic half-lives, and their gastrointestinal absorption efficiency affected by food and medications that suppress gastric acid production. Also, drug-drug interactions can affect antiviral drug plasma levels and affect consistent HIV suppression even with good adherence to the ART regimen. To address these issues and provide individualized guidance, we need studies that include the variety of available treatments, individual subjects' mutation histories, accurate measurement of adherence, and narrow viral load testing intervals.

Although a few studies helped with some initial recommendations, they were designed to better define the links between medication adherence and durability of viral suppression regarding development of resistance and treatment failure. They were not designed to define ideal monitoring intervals for ensuring no viral transmission. As a further limitation, these studies were conducted between 2000 and 2011, when most regimens were more complex or demanding and some were less potent than those available at this writing. During 2005–2011, Benator et al. followed 791 patients from the Washington, D.C., Veterans Affairs Medical Center who had 2 consecutive viral loads below the lower limits of quantitation (LLOQ) within 390 days, followed by at least 1 subsequent viral load. More than half (55%) experienced viral rebound, defined as a viral load greater than the LLOQ. Most of these patients (77%) had at least 1 viral load that exceeded 200 copies/mL, and the likelihood of this level of viral rebound was greatest in the first 3 years of treatment and was related to CD4 count at initiation of ART. Those whose initial CD4 count was less than 300 cells/µL were twice as likely (40% vs. 20%) as those whose initial CD4 was 300 cells/µL or greater to experience viral rebound to greater than 200 copies/mL. Although the rates steadily declined for each group, there remained a difference between the 2 until 6–7 years when the rates converged and became 0.

Lima et al. followed 1305 antiretroviral naïve Canadian patients between January 2000 and June 2007 who had at least 2 consecutive viral loads less than 50 copies/mL after initiation of treatment. Only 274 (21%) of these individuals subsequently experienced viral rebound. The median time of suppression before rebound was 2 years (interquartile range [IQR] 1.1–3.5 years). Their protocol required viral load testing at baseline, 4 weeks after initiation of ART, and quarterly thereafter. The longer the duration of suppression was, the less likely was viral rebound. After adjusting for duration of suppression, those subjects whose adherence was less than 95%

were 11% more likely to rebound than those whose adherence was 95% or greater. Subjects whose virus had drug resistance were 2.78 times more likely to experience viral rebound than those with no resistance. Although the investigators found that while adherence was very important in the first year, the longer suppression was maintained, the less critical adherence became.

A study from the UK Collaborative HIV Cohort, which followed 16,101 patients starting their first regimen between 1998 and mid-2013, also supported the concept that rate of viral rebound declines over time until about 7 years from baseline and then remains very low (about 2.5 per 100 person-years in this study) thereafter.

Regarding the speed of viral control, an important new study employed mathematical modeling to estimate HIV transmission events during the first 8 weeks after initiation of ART. The investigators used HIV-1 RNA decay modeled from the databases of three clinical trials that compared regimens containing the integrase strand inhibitor (INSTI) dolutegravir (DTG) to regimens containing another INSTI, raltegravir (RAL); the non-nucleoside reverse transcriptase inhibitor (NNRTI) efavirenz (EFV); or the protease inhibitor (PI) darunavir/ritonavir (DRV/r). All regimens substantially reduced transmission from the expected number with no treatment. During the 8 weeks following ART initiation, DTG or RAL regimens reduced simulated HIV-1 transmission events by 99.90%. By contrast, EFV and DRV/r reduced simulated transmission events by 76% and 60%, respectively. Although this modeling study is not a clinical trial, it is based on serial viral load measurements within 3 clinical trials and on behavioral risk questionnaires from another large clinical trial.

HOW SHOULD WE COUNSEL OUR PATIENTS?

Where does all of this leave us in the U = U era? We know that if HIV viral load is consistently held to replication levels below 200 copies/mL, there is no sexual transmission of virus. We do not know precisely how many consecutive quarterly viral load measurements should be done to ensure durable suppression, but suppression should not be assumed until a minimum of 2 consecutive measurements taken 3 months apart are below 50 copies/mL. We do not know what to recommend for those individuals whose viral loads do not rapidly fall below 50 copies/mL as we have come to expect with the newer integrase-based regimens. Although the INSTI-containing regimens appeared to result in shorter time to initial viral suppression, we still need more evidence for consistent suppression during that first 6 months to 1 year. Until more data are presented, it seems prudent to recommend that sexual partners of individuals living with HIV who are highly adherent to treatment use PrEP for at least the first 6 months to 1 year following initiation of HIV treatment, and that viral load testing be performed quarterly for at least the first 2 years in the partner living with HIV.

Recommendations regarding PrEP use for the individual not living with HIV should be based on the totality of their risk for HIV exposure, not just within a steady serodiscordant relationship. Are there outside partners? How well do the serodiscordant partners know one another? It is likely there will be different dynamics between serodiscordant partners depending on a variety of things, such as duration of the relationship, age of the partners, and degree of trust. These will influence decisions about forgoing barrier protection and PrEP once the HIV-infected partner has reached consistent viral suppression.

In conclusion, U = U is the scientific maxim that supports treatment as prevention; it removes stigma and permits sexual intimacy and reproduction free from fear of HIV transmission. However, it remains vital that individuals living with HIV remain fully engaged in medical care and that medical providers have the best evidence with which to counsel their patients.

KEY POINTS TO REMEMBER

- PrEP use for the individual not living with HIV should be based on the totality of their risk for HIV exposure.
- PrEP use for the individual not living with HIV should continue for 6 months to 1 year after a sexual partner living with HIV starts and is consistently adherent to ART.
- HIV viral load testing should be performed quarterly for at least the first 2 years after ART initiation in the partner living with HIV.
- When possible, an INSTI-based regimen should be used as ART.

Further Reading

Bavinton BR, Pinto AN, Phanuphak N, et al.; Opposites Attract Study Group. Viral suppression and HIV transmission in serodiscordant male couples: an international, prospective, observational, cohort study. *Lancet HIV*. 2018;5(8):e438–e447.

Benator DA, Elmi A, Rodriguez MD, et al. True durability: HIV virologic suppression in an urban clinic and implications for timing of intensive adherence efforts and viral load monitoring. *AIDS Behav*. 2015;19(4):594–600.

Berenguer J, Parrondo J, Landovitz RJ. Mathematical modeling of HIV-1 transmission risk from condomless anal intercourse in HIV-infected MSM by the type of initial ART. *PLoS One*. 2019;14(7):e0219802.

Centers for Disease Control and Prevention. Update: Trends in AIDS Incidence—United States, 1996. *MMWR Morb Mortal Wkly Rep*. 1997;46(37):861–867.

Cohen MS, Chen YQ, McCauley M, et al. Prevention of HIV-1 infection with early antiretroviral therapy. *N Engl J Med*. 2011;365(6):493–505.

Connor EM, Sperling RS, Gelber R, et al.; for the Pediatric AIDS Clinical Trials Group Protocol 076 Study Group. Reduction of maternal-infant transmission of human immunodeficiency virus type 1 with zidovudine treatment. Pediatric AIDS Clinical Trials Group Protocol 076 Study Group. *N Engl J Med*. 1994;331(18):1173–1180.

Eisinger RW, Dieffenbach CW, A.S. Fauci AS. HIV viral load and transmissibility of HIV infection: undetectable equals untransmittable. *JAMA*. 2019;321(5):451–452.

Eron JJ, Benoit SL, Jemsek J, et al. Treatment with lamivudine, zidovudine, or both in HIV-positive patients with 200 to 500 CD4+ cells per cubic millimeter. North American HIV Working Party. *N Engl J Med*. 1995;333(25):1662–1669.

Fischl MA, Stanley K, Collier AC, et al. Combination and monotherapy with zidovudine and zalcitabine in patients with advanced HIV disease. The NIAID AIDS Clinical Trials Group. *Ann Intern Med*. 1995;122(1):24–32.

Hamlyn E, Ewings FM, Porter K, et al.; and for the INSIGHT SMART and SPARTAC Investigators. Plasma HIV viral rebound following protocol-indicated cessation of ART commenced in primary and chronic HIV infection. *PLoS One*. 2012;7(8):e43754.

Ho DD, Moudgil T, Alam M. Quantitation of human immunodeficiency virus type 1 in the blood of infected persons. *N Engl J Med*. 1989;321(24):1621–1625.

Larder BA, Darby G, Richman DD. HIV with reduced sensitivity to zidovudine (AZT) isolated during prolonged therapy. *Science*. 1989;243(4899):1731–1734.

Lima VD, Bangsberg DR, Harrigan PR, et al. Risk of viral failure declines with duration of suppression on highly active antiretroviral therapy irrespective of adherence level. *J Acquir Immune Defic Syndr*. 2010;55(4):460–465.

McLeod GX, Hammer SM. Zidovudine: five years later. *Ann Intern Med*. 1992;117(6):487–501.

Musicco M, Lazzarin A, Nicolosi A, et al. Antiretroviral treatment of men infected with human immunodeficiency virus type 1 reduces the incidence of heterosexual transmission. Italian Study Group on HIV Heterosexual Transmission. *Arch Intern Med.* 1994;154(17):1971–1976.

O'Connor J, Smith C, Lampe FC, et al.; UK Collaborative HIV Cohort (CHIC) Study. Durability of viral suppression with first-line antiretroviral therapy in patients with HIV in the UK: an observational cohort study. *Lancet HIV.* 2017;4(7):e295–e302.

Prevention Access Campaign. Home page. https://www.preventionaccess.org/

Quinn TC, Wawer MJ, Sewankambo N, et al. Viral load and heterosexual transmission of human immunodeficiency virus type 1. Rakai Project Study Group. *N Engl J Med.* 2000;342(13):921–929.

Rodger AJ, Cambiano V, Bruun T, et al.; for the PARTNER Study Group. Risk of HIV transmission through condomless sex in serodifferent gay couples with the HIV-positive partner taking suppressive antiretroviral therapy (PARTNER): final results of a multicentre, prospective, observational study. *Lancet.* 2019;393(10189):2428–2438.

Rodger AJ, Cambiano V, Bruun T, et al.; PARTNER Study Group. Sexual activity without condoms and risk of HIV transmission in serodifferent couples when the HIV-positive partner is using suppressive antiretroviral therapy. *JAMA.* 2016;316(2):171–181.

Rodger AJ, Lampe FC, Grulich AE, et al.; International Network for Strategic Initiatives in Global HIV Trials (INSIGHT) START Study Group. Transmission risk behaviour at enrolment in participants in the INSIGHT Strategic Timing of AntiRetroviral Treatment (START) trial. *HIV Med.* 2015;16(suppl 1):64–76.

Vernazza P, Hirschel B, Bernasconi E, Flepp M. HIV transmission under highly active antiretroviral therapy. *Lancet.* 2008;372(9652):1806–1807; author reply 1807.

7 "My doctor changed my HIV medications, and now my hepatitis B is back"

Jessica A. Meisner and Mamta K. Jain

A 45-year-old male with HIV, chronic hepatitis B virus (HBV), hypertension, and alcohol use disorder comes into your office after a recent switch of his HIV medications. Eight months ago, he had a relapse of his alcohol use and frequently began missing doses of his elvitegravir/cobicistat/emtricitabine (FTC)/tenofovir alafenamide (TAF). He had an increase in his viral load from less than 20 copies/mL to 4000 copies/mL and ultimately was found to have developed a K65R mutation. You switched him 4 months ago to dolutegravir (DTG)/abacavir (ABC)/lamivudine (3TC), and he has been virally suppressed since that time, including his viral load 1 week ago. His laboratory test values also showed a CD4 of 190, stable complete blood count and creatinine, but an increase in his liver function tests (LFTs). His alanine transferase (ALT) was 300 IU/L, and aspartate transferase (AST) was 420 IU/L. His current medications include DTG/ABC/3TC, sulfamethoxazole/trimethoprim, injectable naltrexone, and lisinopril.

What Do You Do Now?

MANAGEMENT OF HBV CO-INFECTION

The prevalence of abnormal LFTs varies from 20% to 93% in persons living with HIV (PLWH), but is higher than in the general population. The incidence of abnormal LFTs has been reported as 3.9 cases per 100 person-years, defined as 2 consecutive LFTs above the upper limit of normal. Another study found an incidence of grade 3 or higher liver enzyme elevation was 17.71 per 100 person-years for treatment-naïve and 8.22 per 100 person-years in treatment-experienced patients. This variation is due to (1) different definitions of abnormal LFTs and (2) different risk factors by regions, settings, and exposure. According to the American College of Gastroenterology, the definition of an abnormal LFT is greater than 33 units/L for men or greater than 25 units/L for women.

As a clinician, it is important to think of different causes of abnormal LFTs in PLWH. Table 7.1 outlines different etiologies by infectious causes (viral, fungal, mycobacterial) and noninfectious causes. Noninfectious causes of abnormal LFTs include drug-induced liver injury (DILI), which may be from intentional or unintentional acetaminophen overdose, sulfamethoxazole/trimethoprim, azole, statins, amoxicillin/clavulanic, and other prescribed medication. Information on hepatotoxic medications can be found on at LiverTox (https://www.ncbi.nlm.nih.gov/books/NBK547852/). Some HIV medications have also been associated with DILI, including ritonavir at high doses, other boosted protease inhibitors, and nonnucleoside transcript inhibitors such as efavirenz and nevirapine. Stavudine and didanosine, two medications that are no longer used, have been associated with hepatotoxicity due to mitochondrial damage. Most of the time, removal of the offending agent leads to improvement in LFTs; however, damage from mitochondrial toxicity may not be reversible. A thorough history of medications, including nonprescribed medications, should be obtained, including ingestion of acetaminophen, herbal remedies, and supplements.

Alcoholic liver disease (ALD) is a prevalent cause of abnormal LFTs. Abnormal LFTs will typically show an AST:ALT ratio of at least 2:1 in ALD, with values almost never above 300 IU/L. Ultrasound findings will often show hepatic steatosis, which over time can develop into fibrosis/cirrhosis. It is important to obtain a detailed alcohol use history as the prevalence of any alcohol use in PLWH is 40%, with 11% having hazardous use.

TABLE 7.1   Etiology of Abnormal Liver Function Tests

Etiology	Pattern	Epidemiology	Tests
Viral			
Hepatitis C	ALT>AST	Injection Drug Use, MSM, unregulated tattoos, exposure to blood productions	Hepatitis C Ab reflexed to HCV RNA
Hepatitis B		MSM, injection drug use, multiple sexual partners; birth in endemic country; exposure to blood products	Hepatitis B surface Antigen, Hepatits B core antibody, hepatitis B surface antibody; hepatitis B IgM (in acute and may be positive in flare;
Hepatitis D		Superinfection in those with hepatitis B	check Hepatitis D Ab and viral load
Hepatitis A		Travel to endemic regions; homeless; illicit drug users	Hepatitis A IgG
Hepatitis E		Travel to endemic region; wild meats, farm exposure	Hepatitis E IgG
CMV		consider for acute infection or CD4 <50 cells μ/L	CMV Antibodies, CMV Viral load
Epstein Barr Virus		consider for acute infection or CD4 <50 cells μ/L	EBV antibodies

Continued

TABLE 7.1 **Continued**

Etiology	Pattern	Epidemiology	Tests
Herpes Simplex			HSV PCR
Varicella Zoster Virus			VZV PCR
HIV		Acute HIV	HIV test
Mycobacteria			
MAI		Seen in patients with low CD4	AFB cultures; biopsy
TB		From endemic country, TB risk factors (homeless, incarceration, exposure)	AFB cultures; biopsy
Fungal			
cryptococcus		Seen in patients with low CD4	test for Cryptococcus antigen, biopsy
PJP		Seen in patients with low CD4	biopsy
Histoplasmosis		From endemic area	Urine Histoplasmosis Antigen, biopsy
Bartonella		Cat exposure	Anti-Bartonella, biopsy
Microsporidia		Seen in patients with low CD4	Culture
Non-Infectious			
NAFLD			Ultrasound; biopsy
Alcohol	AST:ALT >2:1		thorough history
Medication induced			thorough history
Recreational drugs			thorough history

TABLE 7.1 **Continued**

Etiology	Pattern	Epidemiology	Tests
Cancer			
Lymphoma			biopsy
Kaposi's Sarcoma		Infection with HHV-8	biopsy
Hepatocellular Cancer		Increased risk among those with underlying cirrhosis	quadruple phase MRI

This can be done by asking, "When was the last time you drank?" "How much did you drink that time?" "How often do you drink in 1 week?" Patients should be counseled on complete cessation of alcohol if there are signs of ALD.

Nonalcoholic fatty liver disease (NAFLD) is increasing in prevalence. NAFLD is due to fat in the liver and is commonly seen in patients with obesity, diabetes mellitus, hyperlipidemia, and metabolic syndromes. In PLWH, NAFLD prevalence is estimated to be around 35%. Nonalcoholic steatohepatitis (NASH) is due to fat buildup in the liver, which causes inflammation and overtime fibrosis. Those with NAFLD can develop NASH and cirrhosis. You do not see the same AST:ALT ratio that you see in ALD, but LFTs are also rarely above 300 IU/L.

Recreational drugs can also lead to abnormal LFTs. It has been reported that amphetamine-type stimulants, especially Ecstasy, can cause acute liver injury, even acute liver failure. Cocaine use can lead to abnormal LFTs as well as more severe liver injury.

Cancers, including lymphoma, Kaposi's sarcoma, and hepatocellular cancer, have also been associated with abnormal LFTs. This is another reason why abnormal LFTs should always prompt evaluation by ultrasound.

Infectious causes of abnormal LFTs include the following: acute and chronic viral hepatitis (hepatitis A virus [HAV]; HBV; hepatitis C virus [HCV]; hepatitis D [in those with hepatitis B]; and hepatitis E); acute HIV; cytomegalovirus (CMV); Epstein-Barr virus (EBV); herpes simplex virus (HSV); and varicella zoster virus (VZV), as well as other organisms, such as *Mycobacterium avium-intracellulare* (MAI) and histoplasmosis, among others.

Any patient with an ALT or AST greater than 5 to 10 times the upper limit of normal should prompt a workup of acute viral hepatitis A, B, and C. The prevalence of chronic HCV in PLWH patients is 20%–30% but can be much higher if the patient has a history of injection drug use. Those with chronic hepatitis C may have normal to slightly elevated liver enzymes. All PLWH should be screened for HCV, and annual screening should be performed for those with ongoing drug use or men who have sex with men.

Hepatitis A is another virus that has been decreasing in incidence due to vaccination, but recently outbreaks have occurred among homeless individuals and those who use illicit drugs. The Advisory Committee on Immunization Practices (ACIP) recommends hepatitis A vaccination for anyone experiencing homelessness. Hepatitis E is a rare cause of acute viral hepatitis and should be considered in those who travel to endemic, areas but cases of acute hepatitis E have also been seen in the United States. Chronic hepatitis E virus can occur in those who are immune suppressed, such as transplant recipients and those with HIV.

Herpesviruses are another infectious cause of abnormal LFTs. CMV and EBV are both herpesviruses that often cause a mononucleosis like illness. An acute infection of either CMV or EBV can often have abnormal LFTs. CMV reactivation is often considered an opportunistic infection in PLWH. However, it is important to consider in patients with CD4 T-cell count less than 50 cells/µL. HSV can cause hepatitis when the disease is disseminated. HSV hepatitis is rare but can lead to fulminant disease. VZV can cause localized skin lesion but can also be disseminated, and if involving the liver can be fatal. Histoplasmosis in a PLWH often manifests as disseminated disease and can cause a granulomatous hepatitis. See Table 7.1 for a more expansive list of infectious causes of abnormal LFTs.

In this patient, a new HIV regimen was started, and DILI should be considered. Abacavir has been associated with LFT abnormality in the setting of a person who is HLA-B5701 positive, but there are rare cases of toxicity in those who are HLA-B701 negative. Integrase inhibitors are generally considered safe, but rare cases of DTG-associated hepatotoxicity has been reported.

In this patient, TAF was discontinued due to a K65R mutation, but the patient had previously been diagnosed with hepatitis B. Prior to withdrawing TAF and FTC, it would have been advisable to recheck HBsAg (hepatitis B surface antigen), HBV DNA, HBeAg (hepatitis B e-antigen), anti-HBe (hepatitis B e antibody), and anti-HBs, to determine if the patient had lost HBsAg and gained anti-HBs, in which case withdrawal of HBV-active tenofovir (either tenofovir disoproxil fumarate [TDF] or TAF) and FTC would not be problematic. There have been rare cases of severe immune suppression due to HIV in which those who are HBsAg negative, anti-HBcore positive, anti-HBs positive who lose anti-HBs and become HBsAg positive, a phenomenon known as reverse seroconversion. It is possible that remaining on TDF- or TAF-based regimens could prevent reverse seroconversion. However, this patient likely has HBsAg-positive, elevated HBV DNA that was being suppressed by TAF and FTC.

In any new PLWH, it is important to screen for HBsAg, anti-HBcore, and anti-HBs. If HBsAg positive, then obtain HBeAg, anti-HBe, and HBV DNA. Patients with an isolated HBcAb (hepatitis B core antibody) have either resolved their infection or could be acutely infected. Occult HBV, defined as HBsAg negative and HBV DNA positive, can occur in 5% to 15% of patients, but its clinical significance is unclear. HBV viremia is low, and liver disease progression is not seen. HBeAg-positive patients have on-going replication and are more likely to rebound if active medications are stopped. HIV patients with hepatitis B (HBsAg positive) should have HBV DNA checked at least 2 times a year. Studies indicated that HIV providers infrequently monitor for hepatitis B serologies or HBV DNA in HIV/HBV co-infected patients. Failure to monitor suppression to both HIV and HBV can lead to inadvertent withdrawal of treatment for HBV, leading to HBV flares, liver failure, need for liver transplant, and even death.

Hepatitis delta virus (HDV) can infect those who are HBsAg positive. The prevalence of HDV in HIV in Europe and North America is 5% to 15%; however, the rates may be higher in those from endemic areas and injection drug users. All PLWH who are HBsAg positive should also be screened for HDV serology. If anti-HDV is positive, then they should have HDV RNA testing. Those with stable chronic HBV who experience worsening of disease (increase in LFTs, decompensation, etc.) should be tested for HDV to look for superinfection.

HIV guidelines recommend using a combination of FTC/TDF or FTC/TAF. To date, there has been no HBV resistance to either TDF or TAF. It is not recommended to be on regimens containing lamivudine alone as resistance to lamivudine will develop within a few years. If a patient cannot be on a TDF- or TAF-containing regimen, entecavir is an option for HBV treatment, but it must be used in combination with a fully active antiretroviral therapy (ART) regimen to treat HIV. Entecavir should never be used in patients with HBV lamivudine resistance or those not on HIV treatment, as resistance to HIV can develop with an M184 mutation. Entecavir should only be used in PLWH if they are on a fully suppressive antiretroviral regimen. Once on treatment, HBV DNA should be monitored every 6 months to monitor for suppression. Although tenofovir resistance has not been reported, it is important to monitor for HBV suppression indefinitely. Patients should have at least a 2 log decrease in their HBV DNA after 6 months. Data suggest that incomplete HBV suppression at 1 year of treatment can occur due to high HBV DNA at baseline and HIV viremia. Even among those with HIV suppression, almost 40% may have incomplete HBV suppression. Another study found median time to HBV DNA suppression was 17 months among those who are 3TC naïve and 50 months among those with prior 3TC exposure. Resistance testing should be sent only in specific circumstances, such as persistent viremia or breakthrough on a treatment regimen (>10-fold increase). Resistance testing can be done by direct sequencing or reverse hybridization performed via commercial resistance assays.

Patients with chronic HBV infection should also be evaluated for fibrosis. Methods to assess fibrosis include liver biopsy, which may be considered a gold standard but it is not utilized frequently due to cost and invasiveness of procedure. Noninvasive tests include FibroScan, ultrasound, or magnetic resonance imaging elastography, Fibrosis-4 (FIB-4), AST to Platelet Ratio Index (APRI), Forns Index, as well as commercial assays such as Hepascore or FibroMeter. Noninvasive methods that utilize AST and ALT values such as Fib-4 or APRI may be inaccurate in staging fibrosis if the patient is already on ART as ALT and AST levels will be lower. Combination testing may increase accuracy of staging. All patients who have cirrhosis should be screened for hepatocellular carcinoma (HCC) with ultrasound every 6 months. Those without cirrhosis should be screened regularly if they have the following risk factors: active hepatitis (elevated ALT, high HBV DNA of > 100,000 copies/mL); family history of HCC; Asian male older than 40 years; Asian female older than 50 years; or Africans/African Americans.

Once HBV DNA is suppressed, then you should check HBeAg to determine if HBeAg seroconversion has occurred. With tenofovir treatment, those who are HBeAg positive will suppress HBV DNA and may seroconvert to HBeAg negative and develop anti-HBe (Figure 7.1).

HIV/HBV co-infected patients can experience immune reconstitution with marked increase in LFTs. Often, the elevation in LFTs is associated with a change in CD4 count, such that a larger change in CD4 cell count leads to a higher increase in LFTs. Confusion may arise on continuing ART or stopping. If elevated LFTs are due to immune reconstitution, continuing ART may be beneficial as this LFT elevation indicates the body's immune system is trying to clear the infection. Elevated LFTs due to DILI would be an indication to stop an offending agent such as ART if it was thought to be the causative agent for DILI. Changes in CD4 count or evidence of hypersensitivity may give clues to which mechanism is likely occurring.

Those who are HBsAg negative and anti-HBs negative, including those who are isolated anti-HBc (Hepatitis B core IgG antibody) positive, should be vaccinated for HBV (Figure 7.1). Clinical trials and observational studies

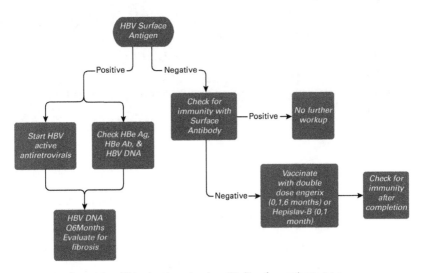

FIGURE 7.1   Approach to HIV patient based on hepatitis B surface antigen status

have shown response rates of 34% to 88% and 34% to 47%, respectively, with 20 μg. Others have examined a 40-μg dose and found 47% responded in a clinical trial and 68% in an observational study. A new hepatitis B recombinant, adjuvanted vaccine is available for prevention. Heplisav-B° (HepB-CpG) is a two-dose series given at baseline and 1 month; it showed superiority compared to the three-dose series of Engerix-B. Although studies in PLWH are not currently available, the ACIP recommends the use of this vaccine for all patients. Factors associated with response included higher CD4 cell count, lower HIV viral load, receipt of ART, female gender, and younger age. It is recommended after completing a vaccination series that anti-HBs should be checked 1–2 months after the series is completed to determine if response occurred. These patients should also be vaccinated against hepatitis A if not already immune.

KEY POINTS TO REMEMBER

- Abnormal LFTs in a patient with HIV require a thorough workup, including review of medications, history, laboratory evaluation, and often an ultrasound.
- Patients with HIV who are HBsAg positive should be evaluated for HBeAg, anti-HBe, and HBV DNA.
- Recommendations are that patients should be placed on a regimen containing TDF or TAF to treat both the HIV and HBV
- Patients should never be placed on lamivudine or entecavir alone to treat their HBV.
- HBV DNA should be monitored every 6 months to asses for suppression.

Further Reading

Benhamou Y, Bochet M, Thibault V, et al. Long-term incidence of hepatitis B virus resistance to lamivudine in human immunodeficiency virus–infected patients. *Hepatology*. 1999;30:1302–1306. doi:10.1002/hep.510300525

Cai J, Osikowicz M, Sebastiani G. Clinical significance of elevated liver transaminases in HIV-infected patients. *AIDS*. 2019;33(8):1267–1282.

Panel on Antiretroviral Guidelines for Adults and Adolescents. Guidelines for the use of antiretroviral agents in adults and adolescents living with HIV. Department of Health and Human Services. 2019 http://www.aidsinfo.nih.gov/ContentFiles/.

Petty LA, Steinbeck JL, Pursell K, Jensen DM. Human immunodeficiency virus and coinfection with hepatitis B and C. *Infect Dis Clin.* 2014;28(3):P477–P499.

Singh KP, Crane M, Audsley J, Avihingsanon A, Sasadeusz J, Lewin SR. HIV-hepatitis B virus coinfection: epidemiology, pathogenesis, and treatment. *AIDS.* 2017;31(5):2035–2052.

8 "I've got HIV and I want to have a baby"

Thana Khawcharoenporn and Beverly E. Sha

A 25-year-old woman was referred from her prenatal care clinic to establish HIV care. This is her first pregnancy, which was recognized by self-testing 8 months ago after missed menstruation. Given her busy work schedule, she had not established prenatal care until this visit. HIV infection was confirmed at the prenatal care clinic. She believes HIV was acquired from her husband, but his status is unknown given no prior testing. The patient denies any underlying comorbidities and current long-term medications. She has been generally healthy. Physical examination reveals normal vital signs. Her history and physical examination are consistent with gestational age of 32 weeks, with an otherwise normal examination. The patient is anxious and expresses concerns about her HIV infection and possibility of transmitting the virus to the baby.

What Do You Do Now?

DISCUSSION

The management of HIV infection among pregnant women has evolved significantly since the introduction of highly effective combination anti-retroviral therapy (ART). The use of ART significantly reduces the risk of perinatal HIV transmission (from 25% to 30% when no intervention is pursued to less than 1% with ART) and increases life expectancy among women living with HIV after delivery. These advances have made it possible for women living with HIV to deliver healthy uninfected infants.

INITIAL EVALUATION AND MANAGEMENT

Ideally, HIV infection is identified prior to pregnancy or as early in pregnancy as possible. This affords the best chance to improve maternal health and prevent maternal-infant HIV transmission. HIV testing of the male partner is also encouraged to assess ongoing risk of HIV acquisition if the woman initially tests negative and to encourage safer sex practices if the couple is serodiscordant (one partner is HIV infected while the other is not HIV infected). Repeat HIV testing in the third trimester prior to 36 weeks' gestation is recommended for pregnant women with initial negative tests if they are at increased risk of acquiring HIV. Third-trimester testing is required in some states based on rates of 1 or more cases per 1000 pregnant women screened and is encouraged for women who are injection drug users, are partners of injection drug users, exchange sex for money or drugs, are sex partners of persons with HIV, have a new sex partner during the pregnancy, are diagnosed with a new sexually transmitted infection (STI) during pregnancy, or have signs or symptoms of acute HIV infection.

Initial evaluation for this pregnant woman should include a through history and physical examination to assess the health of the mother and the fetus. History of comorbid diseases, opportunistic infections (OIs), STIs, drug allergy, medication use, immunization status, and substance abuse should be obtained. The physical examination should assess for signs of advanced HIV infection (i.e., thrush, evidence of wasting or pruritic papular eruption); concomitant STIs (i.e., genital ulcers/lesions, vaginal discharge, or regional lymphadenopathy); and stigmata of chronic liver disease, especially if viral or alcoholic hepatitis is present. Ongoing and modifiable behaviors associated with an increased risk of HIV perinatal transmission such as cigarette smoking, illicit drug use, and genital tract infections should be addressed and discussed with this woman.

Initial laboratory testing should include CD4 cell count to assess for immune status and the need for OI prophylaxis, HIV viral load to assess the virologic response to ART, and HIV drug resistance testing to determine the appropriate ART regimen. HIV ART should be initiated prior to receipt of drug resistance testing results especially for women presenting late in gestation. The initial assessment should also include a complete blood count (CBC); renal and hepatic function testing; testing for viral hepatitis A, B, and C (anti-HAV [hepatitis A virus], HBsAg [hepatitis B surface antigen], anti-HBs [hepatitis B surface antibody], anti-HBc [hepatitis B core antibody], and anti-HCV [hepatitis C virus]); STIs (testing for syphilis, gonorrhea, chlamydia, and trichomonas); and other OIs. Routine immunizations during pregnancy, including primary or booster doses of adult-type tetanus and reduced diphtheria toxoids with pertussis given during each pregnancy at 27–36 weeks' gestation and annual inactivated influenza. Hepatitis A, hepatitis B, and pneumococcal vaccines should be given to this woman if indicated. In addition, she should receive an influenza vaccine during influenza season since both HIV-infected individuals and pregnant women are at risk for severe influenza illness and complications. If the CD4 cell count of this woman is less than 200 cells/μL, prophylaxis with trimethoprim-sulfamethoxazole (TMP-SMX) is warranted for prevention of *Pneumocystis* pneumonia (PCP) (caused by *Pneumocystis jirovecii*) and reactivation toxoplasmosis (if toxoplasma seropositive and CD4 < 100 cells/μL). Alternatives for those with allergies or intolerance to TMP-SMX include dapsone (for PCP) and dapsone with pyrimethamine and leucovorin (for toxoplasmosis).

A first-trimester ultrasound is recommended to confirm gestational age. In this case, an ultrasound should be done as soon as possible.

ANTIRETROVIRAL THERAPY

Antiretroviral therapy reduces the risk of HIV perinatal transmission and improves maternal health. To minimize the risk of perinatal transmission, it is necessary to achieve HIV virologic suppression as early as possible in pregnancy and maintain suppression at the time of delivery. Effective ART among pregnant women involves a 3-part strategy that includes antepartum ART, intrapartum ART, and infant prophylaxis. Among HIV-infected ART-naïve pregnant women, ART should be initiated as early as possible given that each additional week of ART prior to 28 weeks' gestation corresponded to a 10% reduction in the risk of transmission after adjusting for viral load closest to delivery, mode of delivery, and sex. Thus, ART should be initiated before drug resistance testing results return, and the selection of the ART regimen should be based on the primary HIV resistance rates and type in each region.

Antiretroviral Therapy Selection

The ART regimen selected should take into account the local primary HIV drug resistance rates, efficacy, safety, convenience of drug administration, drug interactions with other concurrent drugs, and individual comorbidities, adherence, and preference. Some agents should not be used in pregnant women given limited data or concerns about efficacy and/or safety. These include tenofovir alafenamide (TAF), bictegravir (BIC), nevirapine (NVP), etravirine (ETR), doravirine (DOR), maraviroc (MVC), fosamprenavir (FPV), tipranavir (TPV), and enfuvirtide (T20). In addition, cobicistat-boosted antiretroviral drugs, such as elvitegravir (EVG)/cobicistat (EVG/c), atazanavir/cobicistat (ATV/c), and darunavir/cobicistat (DRV/c) are not recommended due to lower drug levels in the second and third trimesters and associated risks of virologic failure. The recommended antiretroviral drug regimens and important adverse reactions for pregnant women living with HIV are shown in Table 8.1.

The typical ART regimen comprises 2 backbone agents and a third drug. The recommended backbone agents are tenofovir disoproxil fumarate (TDF) with either emtricitabine (FTC) or lamivudine (3TC) or abacavir (ABC)/3TC. The ABC/3TC backbone requires a negative HLA-B*5701 test to avoid ABC hypersensitivity reactions. TDF/FTC or TDF/3TC are preferred for those with hepatitis B virus co-infection. TDF-based backbones require monitoring of renal function and should not be used in individuals with creatinine clearance less than 30 mL/min. The recommended third drugs are ritonavir-boosted protease inhibitors (PI/rs), including ritonavir-boosted atazanavir (ATV/r) and ritonavir-boosted

TABLE 8.1 Antiretroviral Drug Regimen for Treatment and Prevention of Mother-to-Child HIV Transmission

Population (Purpose)	Antiretroviral Drugs		Adverse Reaction	Comment
	Type	Drug Name		
Pregnant women living with HIV (antenatal treatment)	Dual NRTI backbone	TDF/FTC (FDC)	Decreased eGFR, proximal tubular toxicity, bone density loss, nausea/vomiting, dizziness	Adverse reactions of TDF can be enhanced with concurrent use of boosted PIs.
		TDF + 3TC	TDF: decreased eGFR, proximal tubular toxicity, bone density loss, nausea/vomiting, dizziness 3TC: nausea/vomiting, dizziness, anemia	Adverse reactions of TDF can be enhanced with concurrent use of boosted PIs.
		ABC/3TC (FDC)	Hypersensitivity reaction from ABC, insomnia, nausea, headache, dizziness	HLA-B*5701 test is required prior to initiation. This FDC is not recommended if pretreatment HIV RNA is more than 100,000 copies/mL, unless used with DTG.
		ATV/r	Hyperbilirubinemia, nausea/vomiting, insomnia, dizziness, nephrolithiasis	
		DRV/r	Diarrhea, nausea/vomiting, insomnia	Twice-daily administration is required during pregnancy.
	Third drug INSTI	DTG	Insomnia, headache, dizziness	Available as FDC with ABC/3TC
		RAL	Insomnia, headache, dizziness	Twice-daily administration is required.

Continued

TABLE 8.1 Continued

Population (Purpose)	Antiretroviral Drugs Type	Drug Name	Adverse Reaction	Comment
Pregnant women living with HIV (intrapartum treatment)	ZDV (intravenous)		Nausea/vomiting, myalgia, anemia	For women with HIV RNA > 1000 copies/mL near the time of delivery (add on to baseline ART). Can consider addition for women with near-term HIV RNA 50–999 copies/mL. For women with no antenatal ART.
Infants at low risk for perinatal HIV transmission (prophylaxis)	ZDV for 4 weeks			For infants born to mothers on ART since the first trimester with sustained viral suppression and without other risks for HIV transmission.
Infants at higher risk for perinatal HIV transmission (prophylaxis)	ZDV for 6 weeks and 3 doses of NVP during the first week of life **OR** ZDV for 6 weeks and 3TC and NVP for 2–6 weeks **OR** ZDV for 6 weeks and 3TC and RAL for 2–6 weeks		ZDV: nausea/vomiting, myalgia, anemia 3TC: nausea/vomiting, dizziness, anemia NVP: nausea/vomiting, rashes, hepatitis, dyslipidemia RAL: insomnia, headache, dizziness	For infants born to mothers who have not been on ART or with detectable or unknown HIV RNA status at the time of delivery or with other risks for HIV transmission.

Abbreviations: ABC, abacavir; ART, antiretroviral therapy; ATV/r, ritonavir-boosted atazanavir; DRV/r, ritonavir-boosted darunavir; DTG, dolutegravir; eGFR, estimated glomerular filtration rate; FDC, fixed-dose combination; FTC, emtricitabine; HIV, human immunodeficiency virus; INSTI, integrase strand transfer inhibitor; NVP, nevirapine; PI, protease inhibitor; RAL, raltegravir; RNA, ribonucleic acid; 3TC, lamivudine; TDF, tenofovir disoproxil fumarate; ZDV, zidovudine.

[a] According to the Department of Health and Human Services (HHS) Panel on Treatment of HIV-Infected Pregnant Women and Prevention of Perinatal Transmission. Recommendations for use of antiretroviral drugs in pregnant HIV-1-infected women and interventions to reduce perinatal HIV transmission in the United States. https://aidsinfo.nih.gov/contentfiles/lvguidelines/perinatalgl.pdf

darunavir (DRV/r) or integrase strand transfer inhibitors (INSTIs), including dolutegravir (DTG) and raltegravir (RAL).

Recent data from Botswana demonstrated a small increased risk of neural tube defects in infants born to mothers who were on DTG at the time of conception, 0.3% (5 of 1683 on DTG) versus 0.1% (15 of 14,792 on any non-DTG ART). Balancing this information against the higher rates and faster virologic suppression and higher genetic barrier to resistance of DTG compared to other antiretroviral agents, in December 2019, the US Department of Health and Human Services Panel moved DTG back to a preferred antiretroviral throughout pregnancy. For women trying to conceive, DTG is an alternative drug.

If ART is initiated after the first trimester, an INSTI is preferable to a PI/r as the third drug due to the more rapid HIV virologic suppression, especially in pregnant women living with HIV who present for prenatal care in the third trimester like this woman. Alternative backbone drugs for those who cannot take the recommended ones are zidovudine (AZT)/3TC, which has extensive experience and data for use in perinatal HIV transmission prevention. However, adverse reactions and twice-daily dosing are drawbacks.

Alternatives for the third drug include ritonavir-boosted lopinavir (LPV/r), rilpivirine (RPV), and EFV. However, they are less desirable due to adverse reactions of LPV/r and EFV, while RPV should not be used in those with baseline HIV RNA of more than 100,000 copies/mL and/or CD4 cell count less than 200 cells/μL due to reduced efficacy in these patients.

A recent study conducted among pregnant African women who were initiated ART regimens containing DTG versus EFV at a gestation age of at least 28 weeks demonstrated that a significantly higher proportion of pregnant women receiving DTG achieved virologic suppression at delivery compared to those receiving EFV, while there were no significant differences in adverse events and obstetric complications between the two groups. With the late presentation for antenatal care of this woman, TDF/FTC and DTG are considered to be the most appropriate regimen due to the rapid HIV viral load reduction to achieve virologic suppression at delivery and the once-daily dosing, which can promote adherence to the regimen.

Monitoring After Antiretroviral Therapy

Plasma HIV RNA levels should be rechecked 2–4 weeks after initiating or changing ART, then monthly until undetectable, and then every 3 months during pregnancy. CD4 cell counts are recommended every 3–6 months during pregnancy for women who have been on ART for less than 2 years or have had inconsistent adherence. Monitoring for complications of ART with a CBC or renal/liver function tests should be based on the expected toxicity of the specific ART given. After ART initiation, the rate of virologic suppression is expected to be similar between pregnant and nonpregnant women. In one analysis, 93% of the women living with HIV achieved HIV RNA less than 400 copies/mL 3 months after starting ART.

With an INSTI-based regimen, a shorter time to virologic suppression is expected. Detectable viral load at the time of delivery is significantly associated with late initiation of ART and higher HIV transmission rates (0.2%, 0.4%, 0.9%, and 2.2% for ART initiated before conception and during first, second, and third trimesters, respectively). In this woman, 2–3 log reduction in HIV RNA is expected after 1 month of TDF/FTC and DTG. Drug adherence and associated adverse reactions should be monitored closely. Plasma HIV RNA should be reassessed at 36 weeks' gestation to determine mode of delivery. For this woman, if there is an inadequate reduction in viral load at 36 weeks' gestation, adherence should be assessed, and consideration should be given to repeat HIV drug resistance and/or modification of her ART regimen.

INTRAPARTUM MANAGEMENT

Management of pregnant women living with HIV requires discussions on the mode of delivery, minimizing invasive procedures, and use of intrapartum ART.

Mode of Delivery

Pregnant women living with HIV who respond to ART and achieve an HIV RNA of less than 1000 copies/mL near delivery have a low risk of HIV transmission to infants regardless of mode of delivery (elective cesarean section vs. spontaneous vaginal delivery) and duration of membrane rupture. Pregnant women who have not received ART and/or their HIV

RNA near delivery is 1000 copies/mL or greater should undergo elective cesarean section at 38 weeks' gestation since the transmission rate is lower than spontaneous vaginal delivery (8.4% vs. 16.7% in a meta-analysis of 8533 mother-child pairs, of whom 4675 received no ART). In cases with prolonged rupture of membranes and advanced labor, the risk of HIV transmission is comparable between the two modes of delivery.

Intrapartum and Other Interventions

Minimizing the duration of fetal exposure to maternal blood and fluid is crucial to reducing the risk of perinatal HIV transmission. In viremic women, artificial rupture of membranes, use of fetal scalp electrodes, and use of forceps or a vacuum extractor for delivery should be avoided unless there are obstetric indications and the benefits of such procedures outweigh the risk of HIV transmission. If clinically indicated, amniocentesis should be performed when women have undetectable levels.

Intrapartum Antiretroviral Therapy

In general, pregnant women living with HIV should continue their antepartum ART regimen through delivery. Intrapartum intravenous AZT (2 mg/kg loading dose followed by a continuous infusion of 1 mg/kg/h) until delivery is recommended for women with HIV RNA greater than 1000 copies/mL near delivery, poor adherence to ART or no ART during pregnancy, or with unknown HIV RNA quantification. Intravenous AZT should be started 3 hours before elective cesarean delivery. For women with near delivery HIV RNA 50–999 copies/mL, intrapartum intravenous AZT can be considered.

INFANT PROPHYLAXIS

Every infant born to a mother living with HIV should be started on ART within 6–12 hours of the delivery. The recommended regimens are shown in Table 8.1. For those born to a mother who received ART during pregnancy with sustained viral suppression, AZT should be prescribed for 4 weeks. Combination ART is recommended for infants at higher risk of perinatal HIV transmission due to late gestation antenatal ART initiation or detectable maternal HIV RNA near delivery. For these infants (including this case), two-drug combination ART with AZT and 3 prophylactic doses of NVP or three-drug combination ART with AZT/3TC/NVP or RAL for 6 weeks is recommended.

POSTPARTUM MANAGEMENT

Avoidance of breastfeeding is the standard recommendation for women in the United States. After delivery, pregnant women living with HIV should continue lifelong ART with ongoing monitoring. In this case, she can remain on TDF/FTC/DTG unless there is evidence of drug resistance or intolerance or she plans on having another child in the near future.

CONCLUSIONS

In this chapter, we presented the case of a pregnant woman living with HIV with late prenatal care. This case highlights the importance of early care engagement, screening, risk behavior modification, and selection of ART regimens effective in rapidly reducing HIV RNA to achieve virologic suppression at the time of delivery. In addition, close monitoring of virologic response with prompt intervention, appropriate intrapartum management, infant prophylaxis, and counseling are critical to minimize the risk of perinatal HIV transmission among pregnant women living with HIV.

KEY POINTS TO REMEMBER

- Achieving HIV RNA suppression with ART before delivery is a key to reducing perinatal HIV transmission.
- For pregnant women who present late for antenatal care, an INSTI-based regimen is preferred due to shorter time to viral suppression.
- The initial selection of an ART regimen for pregnant women living with HIV should be based on local primary HIV drug resistance rates, efficacy, safety, convenience of drug administration, drug interactions, individual comorbidities, and patient preference.

- Optimal intrapartum management, which includes intrapartum ART, determination of appropriate mode of delivery and minimizing invasive interventions, and infant ART prophylaxis contributes to preventing perinatal HIV transmission.

Further Reading

Committee on Obstetric Practice, HIV Expert Work Group. ACOG committee opinion No. 751: Labor and delivery management of women with human immunodeficiency virus infection. *Obstet Gynecol*. 2018;132:e131–e137.

Department of Health and Human Services (HHS) Panel on Treatment of HIV-Infected Pregnant Women and Prevention of Perinatal Transmission. Recommendations for use of antiretroviral drugs in pregnant HIV-1-infected women and interventions to reduce perinatal HIV transmission in the United States. https://aidsinfo.nih.gov/contentfiles/lvguidelines/perinatalgl.pdf. Accessed 01/18/20.

European AIDS Clinical Society (EACS). Treatment of pregnant women living with HIV, EACS Guidelines, version 10.0. November 2019. https://www.eacsociety.org/files/2019_guidelines-10.0_final.pdf

World Health Organization. Policy brief: update of recommendations on first- and second-line antiretroviral regimens. July 2019. https://www.who.int/hiv/pub/arv/arv-update-2019-policy/en/

Zash R, Holmes L, Diseko M, et al. Neural-tube defects and antiretroviral treatment regimens in Botswana. *N Engl J Med*. 2019;381(9):827–840.

9 "My baby has a fever"

Mariam Aziz

An 8-week-old boy presents with a 3-day history of
fevers, poor feeding, and diarrhea and 1 day of cough.
The infant was born at 38 weeks via cesarean section to
a mother living with HIV. She was started on Epzicom
and raltegravir at week 28 upon prenatal care entry
and at delivery had an HIV-1 RNA of 6400. She was
given intravenous zidovudine intrapartum. The infant's
HIV DNA at birth was negative. The infant completed 6
weeks of antiretroviral therapy (ART) prophylaxis per
mother, but has not been seen for follow-up. The infant
is febrile, tachycardic, tachypneic, and severely hypoxic.
He has a sunken anterior fontanelle, with subcostal
and intercostal retractions, lungs with dry crackles and
wheezing bilaterally and has delayed capillary refill
Neurologic examination showed marked irritability, but
otherwise normal neonatal reflexes. The infant has an
elevated white blood cell count and a low hemoglobin
value. Serum electrolytes and liver and kidney functions
are normal, but lactate dehydrogenase (LDH) is elevated
at 505. A respiratory virus PCR was negative for
respiratory syncytial virus (RSV) and influenza A and B.

What Do You Do Now?

RESPIRATORY ILLNESS IN AN INFANT DIAGNOSED WITH HIV

The infant presented has several concerning aspects. The infant is considered high risk for the acquisition of HIV given the maternal HIV-1 RNA viral load was over 1000 copies/mL at the time of delivery and the mother had started therapy late in pregnancy. Despite cesarean section and neonatal prophylaxis, HIV infection should be considered in this patient. This patient was prescribed combination neonatal prophylaxis, but it is unclear if this was completed as the patient did not undergo routine follow-up HIV testing.

The respiratory symptoms and other systemic illness has a broad differential diagnosis given his immunocompromised status and includes *Pneumocystis jirovecii* pneumonia (PJP; formerly known as *Pneumocystis carinii* pneumonia, PCP), atypical bacterial pneumonia, RSV, influenza virus, parainfluenza viruses, and other opportunistic infections. In children living with HIV, there are 4 clinical variables that are independently associated with PJP; age less than 6 months, respiratory rate greater than 60 breaths per minute, arterial hemoglobin saturation of 92% or less, and the absence of emesis.

Given the broad differential diagnosis, imaging is indicated. A chest x-ray revealed bilateral diffuse parenchymal infiltrates with ground glass or reticulonodular appearance (Figure 9.1). As in adults with HIV, this can be seen in numerous etiologies, including PJP. Given the broad differential, the definitive diagnosis for PJP would be elucidated by sputum obtained by bronchoscopy and bronchoalveolar lavage (BAL). This patient's BAL was sent for PJP immunofluorescent smear and was positive. HIV RNA PCR showed more than 2million copies/mL, and the CD4 count was 620 (Stage 3/AIDS for children less than 1 year old).

By ages 2 to 4 years, more than 80% of children overall will have acquired antibodies to *Pneumocystis*, which is an opportunistic infection seen in children perinatally infected with HIV. Chest x-rays commonly reveal bilateral diffuse parenchymal infiltrates with ground glass or reticulonodular appearance. However, chest x-rays can be normal or only have mild infiltrates. Usually, infiltrates are perihilar but rarely are lobar, cavitary, nodular, or miliary lesions seen. PJP can also be associated pneumothorax or pneumomediastinum. LDH is often increased. Definitive diagnosis is

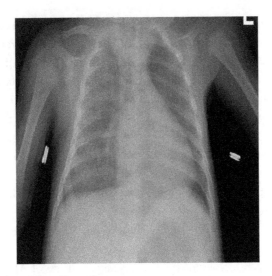

FIGURE 9.1 Infant with respiratory distress

through demonstration of the organism in pulmonary tissues or fluid. A cyst wall, trophozoite, and immunofluorescent antibody stain is recommended for specimens, although immunofluorescent antibody stains are more sensitive and specific than other methods. The Gomori methenamine silver method and toluidine blue stains reveal the cyst wall. Stains such as Giemsa or Wright stains depict the trophozoites but do not stain the cyst wall. While samples can be obtained via nasogastric tube or induced sputum samples in older children, BAL is the procedure of choice, and fluid can remain positive more than 72 hours after start of treatment. First-line therapy is with trimethoprim-sulfamethoxazole. There are no controlled studies for the use of glucocorticoids in children, but most experts would use this as a part of therapy in moderate-to-severe infection.

PEDIATRIC HIV OVERVIEW

The transmission of HIV from a mother living with HIV can happen any time during pregnancy, labor, delivery, or breastfeeding. In resource-rich areas, where breastfeeding is not recommended, pregnancy accounts for 25% to 35% of the transmission, while 65%–75% occurs during labor and delivery. During vaginal delivery, the infant is exposed to virus in the maternal cervicovaginal secretions or blood. The transplacental transmission of HIV is the result of a complex interaction of genetic factors of the mother, the infant, and the virus. However, the predominant risk factor for transmission remains maternal viral load. Without any intervention, transmission rates range from 15% to 45% but can be reduced to less than 2% with interventions during pregnancy or delivery and with neonatal prophylaxis. Maternal risk factors that are associated with in utero infection include maternal drug use during pregnancy, maternal antenatal viral load, delayed start of antiretroviral treatment during pregnancy, and duration of rupture of membranes. Early studies from the Women and Infants Transmission study showed how maternal child transmission varied based on delivery viral load.

The general principles of the pathogenesis and use of ART are similar to adults, but there are some additional considerations in infants and children living with HIV. This is due to the fact that infection has occurred in an immunologically immature individual with rapid growth in the first years of life. Clinical manifestations of HIV in infants and children are often nonspecific. In the first year of life, failure to thrive, recurrent oral candidiasis, and developmental delay are all common presentations. Common AIDS-defining illnesses that are also seen in adults include PJP pneumonia, recurrent bacterial infections, , esophageal candidiasis, disseminated *Mycobacterium avium* complex, or cytomegalovirus infection, among others. Lymphoid interstitial pneumonia was seen more commonly in children than adults prior to the use of combination ART. The World Health Organization (WHO) has criteria for use in the developing world and the Centers for Disease Control and Prevention (CDC) in the United States have developed surveillance case definitions used for monitoring HIV infection based on absolute CD4 T-cell counts and AIDS-defining illness. The CDC criteria are not the basis for clinical decisions in individual patients, while the WHO criteria allow for the initiation of ART based on clinical criteria without results from definitive laboratory testing.

In children, there is a requirement for the use of HIV virologic tests instead of antibody tests to diagnose perinatal HIV infection in infants younger than 18 months of age. In the United States, recommendations are for women living with HIV to refrain from breastfeeding. A definitive

HIV diagnosis can be made in most nonbreastfed infants through the use of virologic assays by 1 month of age and in virtually all nonbreastfed infants by 4 months of age. Transplacental transfer of maternal antibodies precludes the use of HIV antibody testing in infants. These antibodies may be present in infants up to 12–15 months of age, so a virologic test must be used to establish true infection. Virologic tests that can be used include the detection of HIV-1 RNA or proviral DNA. Some experts would suggest that HIV-1 DNA assays are the preferred tests in newborns still receiving antiretroviral prophylaxis.

The Department of Health and Human Services (DHHS) Panel on Antiretroviral Therapy and Medical Management of Children Living with HIV indicates that HIV infection can be presumptively excluded in nonbreastfed infants with 2 or more negative virologic tests (1 obtained at 14 or more days of age, and the other is obtained at 1 month or more of age) or 1 negative virologic test result obtained at 2 months or more of age or 1 negative HIV antibody test result at 6 months of age or older. To definitively exclude HIV infection in these nonbreastfed infants, 2 or more negative virologic tests must be obtained (1 at ≥ 1 month of age and another at ≥ 4 months of age) or 2 negative HIV antibody tests from separate specimens obtained at 6 months or more of age.

HIV infection is confirmed by 2 positive HIV virologic tests performed on separate blood samples, regardless of age. In rare cases, patients may seroconvert up to 24 months of age. Although most infants without HIV infection serorevert by 15–18 months of age, allowing the absence of HIV infection to be confirmed with an HIV antibody test performed at 15–18 months of age or older, late seroreversion (after 18 months of age) can occur. Diagnosis of children who are older than 24 months of age uses standard HIV antibody testing.

There are unique issues related to the treatment of HIV in this patient population. This includes age-specific differences in CD4 count and changes in pharmacokinetic parameters caused by continuing maturation of the organs involved with metabolism of drugs. Interpreting CD4 count and percentages in children must take age into consideration. CD4 counts and percentage values in healthy infants without HIV are considerably higher than adults without HIV. These values slowly decline by age 5 years (Table 9.1). The early management of HIV-exposed infants has been

TABLE 9.1 HIV Infection Stage Based on Age-Specific CD4 Cell Count or Percentage

Stage[a]	Age at the Time of the CD4 Test					
	<1 Year	%	1 Year to <6 Years	%	≥6 Years	%
	Cells/μL		Cells/μL		Cells/μL	
1	≥1,500	≥34	≥1000	≥30	≥500	≥26
2	750–1499	26–33	500–999	22–29	200–499	14–25
3	<750	<26	<500	<22	<200	<14

[a]The stage is based primarily on the CD4 cell count; the CD4 cell count takes precedence over the CD4 percentage, and the percentage is considered only when the count is missing. If a Stage 3–defining condition has been diagnosed, then the stage is 3 regardless of CD4 test results.
Source: Centers for Disease Control and Prevention. Revised surveillance case definition for HIV infection—United States. 2014. *Morb Mortal Wkly Rep.* 2014;63(RR-3):1–10.

rapidly evolving since a case report in 2013 and follow-up papers that have discussed an infant with HIV who was started on combination ART very early (~30 hours of life) and resulted in an apparent functional cure. The infant was on ART until 18 months of age and had an unplanned treatment cessation. The infant had a plasma HIV-1 RNA less than 20 copies through 30 months of age and no HIV-1–specific antibodies at 24, 26, or 28 months of age. After being off of antiretrovirals for almost 2 years, the patient, who was now nearly 4 years old, had detectable virus in the blood and detectable HIV antibodies, likely reflecting true HIV infection at birth with active HIV replication off combination ART from previously latent viral reservoirs.

Given this case and a growing body of literature in this area, in the setting of high risk for mother-to-child transmission, many experts would consider treating the newborn baby with combination ART. Infants are considered high risk if born to mothers who did not receive intrapartum or antepartum antiretroviral agents, mothers who received only intrapartum antiretroviral agents, mothers who received combination ART but did not experience HIV-1 RNA suppression near delivery, or mothers who have primary or acute HIV infection during pregnancy. The current DHHS perinatal guidelines recommend either 2 drugs with 6 weeks of zidovudine and 3 doses of nevirapine (with doses given within 48 hours of birth, 48 hours after first dose, and 96 hours after second dose) versus combination HIV therapy using either/or zidovudine, lamivudine and nevirpaine or zidovudine, lamivudine and raltegravir depending on the gestational age and other birth factors.

To guide future recommendations, there are ongoing clinical trials that are looking at this 3-drug treatment regimen in infants who are high risk or with confirmed HIV. At this time, there are minimal data on antiretrovirals in children less than 6 weeks of age. Treatment guidelines from the DHHS recommend the initiation of ART in children less than 12 months of age regardless of clinical status due to improved outcomes. Factors related to adherence are important to discuss with patients' primary caretakers and family before treatment initiation.

The progression of HIV is much more rapid in children than adults. The Children With HIV Early Antiretroviral Therapy (CHER) study showed 76% reduction in early mortality and 75% reduction in HIV progression when ART was initiated in asymptomatic, perinatally infected children who had CD4 T cells greater than 25% before 12 weeks of age compared to a delayed start based on clinical signs and symptoms and most deaths occurred in the first 6–9 months of life. Other studies have also shown that early use of ART in infants results in improved clinical and immunologic outcomes. Studies from the International Maternal Pediatric Adolescent AIDS Clinical Trials (IMPAACT) network have shown the mortality rate decline to 0.6 per 100 patients per year in resource-rich settings where most patients were on combination antiretrovirals.

Pneumocystis jirovecii pneumonia is a major cause of morbidity and mortality in the first year of life for infants with HIV, so prophylaxis beginning at 4–6 weeks of age is recommended for infants with indeterminate HIV status and for all children living with HIV aged less than 12 months. HIV-infected children ages 1 to less than 6 with CD4 counts below 500 and HIV-infected children 6 years or older with CD4 counts less than 200 cells/mm^3 should also receive prophylaxis. Because HIV infection can be presumptively excluded if virologic tests at both 14–21 days and 1–2 months are negative, most HIV-exposed infants in the United States do not receive PCP prophylaxis.

- HIV infection needs to be considered in an infant who is high risk (specifically born to mothers who did not receive intrapartum or antepartum antiretroviral agents, mothers who received only intrapartum antiretroviral agents, mothers who received combination ART but did not experience HIV-1 RNA suppression near delivery, or mothers who have primary or acute HIV infection during pregnancy.
- The presence of antibodies against HIV is reflective of transplacental transfer of maternal antibodies and does not necessarily mean HIV infection in infants.
- Virologic tests that can be used include the detection of HIV-1 RNA or proviral DNA and are the tests recommended by the US DHHS Panel on Antiretroviral Therapy and Medical Management of Children Living With HIV.
- *Pneumocystis* pneumonia should be considered in the differential diagnosis of a high-risk infant with respiratory distress.
- *Pneumocystis* pneumonia prophylaxis is indicated starting at 4–6 weeks of life in children living with HIV less than 12 months old.

Further Reading

Aboulker JP, Babiker A, Chaix ML, et al. Highly active antiretroviral therapy started in infants under 3 months of age: 72-week follow-up for CD4 cell count, viral load and drug resistance outcome. *AIDS*. 2004;18(2):237–245.

Centers for Disease Control and Prevention. Revised surveillance case definition for HIV infection—United States, 2014. *MMWR Recomm Rep.* 2014;63(RR-03):1–10.

Cooper ER, Charurat M, Mofenson L, et al. Combination antiretroviral strategies for the treatment of pregnant HIV-1-infected women and prevention of perinatal HIV-1 transmission. *J Acquir Immune Defic Syndr.* 2002;29(5):484–494.

Fatti GL, Zar HJ, Swingler GH. Clinical indicators of *Pneumocystis jiroveci* pneumonia (PCP) in South African children infected with the human immunodeficiency virus. *Int J Infect Dis.* 2006;10(4):282–285.

Faye A, Bertone C, Teglas JP, et al. Early multitherapy including a protease inhibitor for human immunodeficiency virus type 1-infected infants. *Pediatr Infect Dis J.* 2002;21(6):518–525.

Faye A, Le Chenadec J, Dollfus C, et al. Early versus deferred antiretroviral multidrug therapy in infants infected with HIV type 1. *Clin Infect Dis.* 2004;39(11):1692–1698.

Luzuriaga K, Gay H, Ziemniak C, et al. Viremic relapse after HIV-1 remission in a perinatally infected child. *N Engl J Med.* 2015;372(8):786–788.

Luzuriaga K, McManus M, Catalina M, et al. Early therapy of vertical human immunodeficiency virus type 1 (HIV-1) infection: control of viral replication and absence of persistent HIV-1-specific immune responses. *J Virol.* 2000;74(15):6984–6991.

Magder LS, Mofenson L, Paul ME, et al. Risk factors for in utero and intrapartum transmission of HIV. *J Acquir Immune Defic Syndr.* 2005;38(1):87–95.

Mirani G, Williams PL, Chernoff M, et al. Changing trends in complications and mortality rates among US youth and young adults with HIV infection in the era of combination antiretroviral therapy. *Clin Infect Dis.* 2015;61(12):1850–1861.

Nielsen-Saines K, Watts DH, Veloso VG, et al. Three postpartum antiretroviral regimens to prevent intrapartum HIV infection. *N Engl J Med.* 2012;366(25):2368–2379.

Panel on Antiretroviral Therapy and Medical Management of Children Living With HIV. Guidelines for the use of antiretroviral agents in pediatric HIV infection. http://aidsinfo.nih.gov/contentfiles/lvguidelines/pediatricguidelines.pdf. Accessed November 1, 2019.

Panel on Opportunistic Infections in HIV-Exposed and HIV-Infected Children. Guidelines for the prevention and treatment of opportunistic infections in HIV-exposed and HIV-infected children. Department of Health and Human Services. http://aidsinfo.nih.gov/contentfiles/lvguidelines/oi_guidelines_pediatrics.pdf. Accessed November 1, 2019.

Panel on Treatment of HIV-Infected Pregnant Women and Prevention of Perinatal Transmission. Recommendations for use of antiretroviral drugs in pregnant HIV-1-infected women for maternal health and interventions to reduce perinatal HIV transmission in the United States. http://aidsinfo.nih.gov/contentfiles/lvguidelines/PerinatalGL.pdf. Accessed November 1, 2019.

Persaud D, Gay H, Ziemniak C, et al. Absence of detectable HIV-1 viremia after treatment cessation in an infant. *N Engl J Med.* 2013;369(19):1828–1835.

Read JS, Committee on Pediatric Aids, American Academy of Pediatrics. Diagnosis of HIV-1 infection in children younger than 18 months in the United States. *Pediatrics.* 2007;120(6):e1547–e1562.

Violari A, Cotton MF, Gibb DM, et al. Early antiretroviral therapy and mortality among HIV-infected infants. *N Engl J Med.* 2008;359(21):2233–2244.

World Health Organization. *WHO Case Definitions of HIV for Surveillance and Revised Clinical Staging and Immunological Classification of HIV-Related Disease in Adults and Children.* Geneva, Switzerland: World Health Organization; 2007.

10 "My hair is falling out, and they told me I have syphilis!"

Ronnie M. Gravett and Jeanne Marrazzo

A 29-year-old male living with HIV on antiretroviral therapy with bictegravir, tenofovir alafenamide, and emtricitabine presents with hair loss for 2 weeks. He reports patchy bald spots on the left side of his head. It does not itch or hurt; there is no redness or scaling. He was diagnosed with HIV 5 years ago by routine screening; he was also diagnosed with and treated for gonorrhea and syphilis at that time. His most recent viral load is undetectable, and his CD4 count is 650 cells/mL^3. He is sexually active with men only, and he reports 4 new partners in the last 3 months. He has oral and anal insertive sex only, and he does not use condoms. Six months ago, at his last checkup, he had positive treponemal antibody and negative rapid plasma reagin (RPR) results. He denies any headache, vision changes, or hearing changes. He has no other symptoms currently. His examination reveals 5-cm patchy alopecia on the left parietal aspect of his head.

What Do You Do Now?

SEXUALLY TRANSMITTED INFECTIONS

This patient's "moth-eaten" hair loss in the setting of multiple new sex partners is suspicious for syphilitic alopecia, a manifestation of secondary syphilis. Although he has a reactive treponemal antibody test, this is likely explained by his prior syphilis diagnosis as that antibody remains reactive indefinitely; the recently nonreactive RPR showed no active infection at that time, but he has had multiple exposures since then. Given the concern for syphilis in this patient, he should have an RPR test repeated now as well as testing for *Chlamydia trachomatis* and *Neisseria gonorrhoeae* (NG) with both urine and extragenital sampling (oropharynx and rectum). Because he is symptomatic and had a recent nonreactive RPR test (<1 year ago), he should be treated for presumed secondary syphilis with 1 dose right now of 2.4 million units of benzathine penicillin by intramuscular injection. He has no neurologic symptoms, and his HIV is well controlled, so there is no need to perform a lumbar puncture at this time. His RPR testing should be repeated in 3 months to assess his general response and in 6 months to ensure adequate, 4-fold decrease in the RPR.

INTRODUCTION

Occurring as a syndemic, HIV and sexually transmitted infections (STIs) are entwined and must be considered in the context of each other. Partitioning these two phenomena into separate HIV and STI silos ignores the interactions at play. STIs significantly burden persons living with HIV (PLWH) at now unprecedented rates. The majority of STIs are actually asymptomatic yet can lead to significant comorbidity without prompt detection and treatment. Routine STI screening of at-risk PLWH, even if asymptomatic, is recommended by national guidelines. This chapter focuses on bacterial STIs affecting PLWH: chlamydia, gonorrhea, and syphilis.

SCREENING

All PLWH who are sexually active should be screened for STIs at least once annually. More frequent screening may be considered based on sexual history, risk assessment, and clinical concerns for STI. Screening should focus on sites with sexual contact, so providers must take a comprehensive sexual health history. As STI rates increase, providers should be particularly mindful to screen at extragenital sites. Chlamydia and gonorrhea screening are accomplished by directly sampling exposed sites, and samples can be self-collected by the patient or clinician collected. Syphilis screening is performed with serology.

CHLAMYDIA

Overview
Chlamydia trachomatis is the most commonly reported STI. It is most often asymptomatic, yet it still causes significant morbidity, particularly as related to reproductive health among women. In 2018, the case report rate was 539.9 cases per 100,000 persons, with a total of nearly 1.8 million reported cases in the United States. Women have the highest case report rate, with 688.2 per 100,000 women. Men who have sex with men (MSM) have seen a sharp increase in chlamydial infections, with an increase in diagnosed infections of 37.8% (as compared to the 11.4% increase among women). Various serovars of the pathogen contribute to disease differently, with serovars L1, L2, and L3 causing lymphogranuloma venereum (LGV) and serovars D–K causing typical oculogenital infections; serovars A–C are responsible for trachoma.

Clinical Features and Diagnosis
Though often asymptomatic among women, chlamydia can cause cervicitis, pelvic inflammatory disease, and chronic pelvic pain. In men, it can cause urethritis or proctitis. LGV is a serious chlamydial syndrome characterized by self-limited ulceration at the site of inoculation and subsequent painful lymphadenopathy, often accompanied by fever and systemic symptoms. Among persons infected through receptive anal intercourse, proctitis is the main manifestation, with significant anal discharge or painful bowel movements.

Diagnosis is best made by a nucleic acid amplification test (NAAT). NAATs are available to test vaginal, cervical, anorectal, and oropharyngeal samples. Culture is available, although not in routine clinical use. If there is clinical concern for LGV, then serotyping is available to identify causative serovars, but treatment for LGV should not be delayed until serovar identification. Screening is recommended for all PLWH at least once annually if sexually active and more frequently depending on their risk.

Treatment

Non-LGV chlamydia can be treated with one oral dose of azithromycin 1000 mg or doxycycline 100 mg orally twice a day (7 days for asymptomatic infection or 21 days for LGV). Doxycycline 100 mg orally may be superior for rectal infections, but data to support this are not conclusive. LGV proctitis requires 21 days of treatment with oral doxycycline (100 mg orally twice daily). Although screening for oropharyngeal chlamydia is not recommended, if detected, then it should be treated. Alternative treatments for chlamydia when azithromycin or doxycycline cannot be used or are unavailable include erythromycin, levofloxacin, or ofloxacin. Follow-up testing following treatment is not recommended.

GONORRHEA

Overview

Gonorrhea, caused by NG, is increasing in incidence, and the continued development of antimicrobial resistance highlights this epidemic. Although frequently asymptomatic, gonorrhea can have varied presentations. MSM have the highest incidence. In 2018, there were 583,405 new cases diagnosed, with a case rate of 179.1 per 100,000 persons, which is more than an 80% increase since 2009, when the number of new cases reached an all-time low.

Clinical Features and Diagnosis

Common manifestations of gonococcal infection among men include urethritis, which is characterized by thick, purulent urethral discharge, usually developing 2–5 days after exposure; epididymitis; prostatitis; and occasionally penile edema. Among women, cervical infection, sometimes with a purulent exudate indicating cervicitis, is common. Rectal infections, particularly among MSM, are increasing significantly and are most often asymptomatic; symptoms, when present, include tenesmus, rectal pain, and mucoid or bloody discharge. Pharyngeal infection is also increasingly common, nearly always asymptomatic, and serves as potential reservoir for transmission. Rarely, gonorrhea can manifest as disseminated gonococcal infection (DGI), resulting from gonococcal bacteremia; DGI includes arthritis-dermatitis syndrome, characterized by asymmetric, polyarticular arthritis (most commonly knees, elbows, and ankles) or tenosynovitis accompanied by papular rash predominantly over the lower extremities.

Diagnosis is best made using NAAT as it is more sensitive than culture; samples may be collected from first-catch urine or swabs obtained from the cervix, urethra, vagina, or oropharynx. Among symptomatic men with purulent urethral exudate, Gram stain showing gram-negative diplococci is very sensitive and specific. Gonorrhea can be cultured using Thayer-Martin media, which allows for antimicrobial susceptibility testing. Antimicrobial resistance is increasing globally; notably, fluoroquinolones are largely considered unusable. Similarly, minimum inhibitory concentrations to third-generation cephalosporins are increasing, although treatment failures in the United States have not yet been reported.

Treatment

Current treatment guidelines recommend dual antimicrobial therapy to compete against emerging antimicrobial resistance. First-line therapy is ceftriaxone 250 mg IM injection once and azithromycin 1000 mg orally once. For cephalosporin-allergic persons, an alternative regimen is dual therapy with either gentamicin 240 mg IM once and oral azithromycin 2000 mg once or oral gemifloxacin 320 mg once and oral azithromycin 2000 mg once. If there is concern for treatment failure, then culture with antibiotic susceptibility testing is appropriate. DGI treatment involves a longer course of therapy and should involve infectious diseases consultation.

SYPHILIS

Overview

Treponema pallidum is the etiologic agent of syphilis. With its protean manifestations, syphilis has long plagued humans. As with other STIs, syphilis is increasing, especially among MSM. In 2018, there were 35,063 new cases of primary or secondary syphilis, a nearly 15% increase from the year prior. MSM currently have the highest burden of infection.

Clinical Features and Diagnosis

Contrary to other STIs, primary and secondary syphilis, by definition, are always symptomatic, but the symptoms may go unrecognized initially. Primary syphilis is characterized by a chancre, typically a painless, indurated ulceration at the site of inoculation. If the ulcer is not directly visualized and is painless, it may go unnoticed until it resolves. Following primary syphilis, secondary syphilis is the dissemination of the spirochete through the body, and it may manifest as a nonspecific illness with fever, malaise, lymphadenopathy, and rash classically involving the palms and soles. A severe and fortunately rare rash, termed *lues maligna*, is seen in persons with advanced, uncontrolled HIV, and it is characterized by persistent ulcerative lesions. Additionally, secondary syphilis can manifest with hair loss, as in the case leading this chapter, oral lesions, condyloma lata, and hepatitis. Asymptomatic syphilis is termed *latent syphilis* and may be described as early (acquired in the past year) or late latent syphilis. Gummas are granulomatous lesions characterizing tertiary syphilis and can affect any tissue or organ, including the brain, bones, and skin.

Neurosyphilis is a complication of syphilis that can occur at any stage, and PLWH may be a higher risk. It should be suspected with any symptoms suggesting central nervous system involvement, such as headache, neck pain, vision or hearing changes, encephalopathy, meningitis, stroke, and cognitive decline. Advanced, long-standing neurosyphilis without treatment can lead to general paresis, a progressive cognitive impairment syndrome, or tabes dorsalis, a demyelinating syndrome affecting posterior columns of the spinal cord and leading to paresthesia, decreased coordination and proprioception, and diminished reflexes.

All stages of syphilis are diagnosed serologically using a sequence of treponemal and nontreponemal tests. Primary and secondary syphilis may be diagnosed microscopically using dark-field microscopy to visualize spirochetes from a clinical sample. Treponemal assays detect antibodies against the organism and indicate prior exposure; after exposure, these assays remain positive. Nontreponemal tests such as the RPR or Venereal

Disease Research Laboratory (VDRL) are serially diluted assays to determine the activity of the syphilis infection. The RPR may be falsely negative in up to 30% of cases of primary syphilis. Extremely high RPR titers may lead to falsely negative tests (the "prozone" effect); in such instances when syphilis is strongly suspected, further dilution will allow for detection by RPR. False-positive RPRs occur not infrequently and may be due to lupus or other autoimmune conditions, pregnancy, and HIV infection; therefore, all reactive RPRs must be confirmed with a treponemal assay. Among persons with prior syphilis, a 4-fold increase in the nontreponemal titer is considered a new infection (or persistence of infection if recently treated).

Neurosyphilis is diagnosed by cerebrospinal fluid (CSF) analysis. The CSF VDRL is very specific but poorly sensitive; therefore, a negative VDRL from the CSF does not rule out syphilis. CSF with elevated white blood cells or elevated protein, in the appropriate clinical context with positive treponemal and nontreponemal tests, should be considered consistent with neurosyphilis and treated empirically. Otic syphilis may often have a relatively normal CSF profile with normal white blood cells and protein and a negative CSF VDRL; if there is clinical concern for auditory or vestibular disease with reactive serologic evaluation for syphilis, then treatment for otic syphilis should be pursued.

Treatment

Optimal therapy for all syphilis stages is penicillin. Primary, secondary, and early latent syphilis should be treated with benzathine penicillin 2.4 million units IM injection once. For late latent, latent of unknown duration, and tertiary syphilis, treatment should be with benzathine penicillin 2.4 million units IM given weekly for 3 weeks, with total dose of 7.2 million units. Neurosyphilis, including ocular and otic syphilis, should be treated with aqueous penicillin G 18–24 million units daily, administered intravenously in 6 divided doses or as a continuous infusion. Table 10.1 shows first-line therapy for bacterial STIs.

Although data for penicillin alternatives are less robust, among penicillin-allergic PLWH with primary or secondary syphilis, oral doxycycline 100 mg twice daily for 14 days may be a reasonable alternative. For these individuals with latent syphilis, oral doxycycline 100 mg twice daily for 28 days may be used with close serologic and clinical follow-up. Patients who are penicillin

TABLE 10.1 **First-Line Treatment for Bacterial STIs**

Organism	Treatment
Chlamydia trachomatis	
Uncomplicated cervical, urethral, or rectal infection:	Azithromycin 1000 mg orally once OR
	Doxycycline 100 mg orally twice daily for 7 days
Lymphogranuloma venereum	Doxycycline 100 mg orally twice daily for 21 days
Neisseria gonorrhoeae	Ceftriaxone 250 mg intramuscularly once AND
	Azithromycin 1000 mg orally once
Treponema pallidum	
Primary, secondary, or early latent syphilis	Benzathine penicillin 2.4 million units IM once
Late latent syphilis	Benzathine penicillin 2.4 million units IM weekly for 3 weeks
or latent of unknown duration	Aqueous penicillin G 18–24 million units IV daily as continuous infusion or 6 divided doses
Neurosyphilis and ocular or otic syphilis	

allergic with neurosyphilis, syphilis while pregnant, or congenital syphilis should undergo penicillin desensitization.

Rarely, as a consequence of treatment, the Jarisch-Herxheimer reaction may occur within the first several hours following treatment, especially among individuals with particularly high titers. Caused by the inflammatory response to killed spirochetes, self-limited symptoms include not only fever, body aches, and headache but also can include chills, rigors, and even hypotension. It may be confused with an allergic reaction to the treatment, but the Jarisch-Herxheimer reaction typically starts a few hours after therapy, as opposed to the much sooner immunoglobulin E–mediated reaction. Patients should be counseled to the possibility of this reaction and treated with nonsteroidal anti-inflammatory agents if it occurs.

Treatment response should be assessed quarterly in PLWH by repeat serology, with the same assay (RPR or VDRL) followed throughout. A 4-fold decrease in serum RPR by 6 months is an appropriate response, with titers expected to be negative by 1 year. If there is not an appropriate decline in titers, then reevaluation for possible neurosyphilis, including CSF analysis, or reinfection should be considered. If there is a 4-fold decline in titers after treatment, but the titers do not revert to nonreactive, then this person may be serofast. No further treatment is indicated in that case.

CONCLUSION

Sexually transmitted infections are very common and often asymptomatic among PLWH. Taking a sexual history, including sexual practices, partners, and symptoms, should be a part of routine care of PLWH. Annual screening for STIs is essential and should be more frequent as determined by sexual history. Prompt treatment can prevent further morbidity and adverse outcomes. Although HIV cannot be transmitted by sexual contact among virally suppressed PLWH, safer sex practices, including emphasized condom use, should be encouraged to help prevent STI acquisition.

KEY POINTS TO REMEMBER

- STIs are increasing to unprecedented levels and occur as a syndemic among PLWH.
- Chlamydia and gonorrhea are often asymptomatic and should be screened routinely using NAATs at sites of exposure.
- After treatment for syphilis, follow-up testing should be quarterly, with an expected 4-fold decline by 6 months; if there is no decline, then consider neurosyphilis reservoir or reinfection.
- Neurosyphilis occurs at any syphilis stage and must be assessed in any PLWH with syphilis and new headache, vision complaints, or other neurologic signs or symptoms.

Further Reading

Aberg JA, Gallant JE, Ghanem KG, Emmanuel P, Zingman BS, Horberg MA. Primary care guidelines for the management of persons infected with HIV: 2013 update by the HIV Medicine Association of the Infectious Diseases Society of America. *Clin Infect Dis.* 2013;58(1):e1–e34.

Centers for Disease Control and Prevention. Sexually transmitted diseases treatment guidelines 2015. *MMWR Recomm Rep*. 2015;64(RR-03):1–137.

Centers for Disease Control and Prevention. *Sexually Transmitted Disease Surveillance 2018*. Atlanta, GA: US Department of Health and Human Services; 2019.

Panel on Antiretroviral Guidelines for Adults and Adolescents. *Guidelines for the Use of Antiretroviral Agents in Adults and Adolescents with HIV*. Atlanta, GA: Department of Health and Human Services. December 18, 2019.

11 "I've been rashed and confused": Part 1

David E. Barker

A 26-year-old man is brought in from a homeless
shelter for altered mental status. Shelter staff reports
that he had only been there for the past few days,
had been more alert when he first arrived, and had
complained of mild shortness of breath, nonproductive
cough, and diarrhea for the past month. The patient
responds slowly and incompletely to questions.

On examination, the patient is cachectic, afebrile, with
normal vital signs. The patient is somnolent, with a Glasgow
coma scale score of 12/15. He has some degree of rigidity,
with downgoing Babinski sign and slightly exaggerated
symmetrical reflexes. Motor strength is intact, with normal
sensation. Examination of the lungs reveals areas of bilateral
crackles.

Admitting laboratory values show a hemoglobin B of 9,
white blood cell count of 5.3, potassium of 2.9, and glucose
of 79. Serum toxicology is negative. Serum syphilis enzyme
immunoassay (EIA) and cryptococcal antigen are negative,
an HIV EIA is positive, and the CD4 count is 11. Noninfused
head computed tomography (CT) shows multiple bilateral
basal ganglia changes, which could represent subacute or
chronic infarction. Cerebrospinal fluid (CSF) is obtained with
an opening pressure of 11 cm, glucose of 30, protein of 80, 1
white blood cell, and 33 red blood cells.

What Do You Do Now?

SUBACUTE DELIRIUM IN AIDS

There are two considerations regarding this patient; the more important is what the cause of the mental status deterioration is; the possibly more immediate one is whether the patient's pulmonary complaint represents tuberculosis (TB), posing a risk to staff.

A chest x-ray is obtained and shows diffuse patchy infiltrates without evidence of adenopathy. A chest CT is then obtained, which demonstrates patches of tree-in-bud opacities, but no dense infiltrates, no adenopathy, and a pattern of involving all lung areas, which would be atypical for *Pneumocystis*. Radiology feels this most likely represents tuberculosis or a fungal infection. Acid-fast bacterial (AFB) and fungal stains of sputum and polymerase chain reaction (PCR) for *Mycobacterium tuberculosis* are negative. A bronchoscopy is performed, and stains for *Pneumocystis jirovecii* pneumonia (PJP), AFB, and fungal organisms are all negative. An AFB blood culture was eventually reported as negative. Urine *Histoplasma* antigen is negative, as is CSF cryptococcal antigen.

On the second hospital day, the patient began to develop focal neurological findings with a slight right facial droop and with decreasing strength in the right upper extremity. The patient remains afebrile.

Magnetic resonance imaging of the brain with contrast is performed, which shows subacute infarcts involving the bilateral posterior parietal lobes as well as bilateral basal ganglia and cerebellar hemispheres. There is also diffuse ependymal contrast enhancement suggestive of ventriculitis.

DIFFERENTIAL

Cryptococci have to be carefully considered in a patient living with AIDS who has subacute mental deterioration and a pulmonary process. However, in contrast to cancer patients, in patients living with AIDS with cryptococcal meningitis, a negative serum antigen test has a very high negative predictive value. The absence of increased opening pressure also weighs strongly against this diagnosis since this condition causes deterioration of mental status, mostly through increased CSF pressure.

Other fungal meningitides, such as with *Histoplasma* or coccidiomycosis, are possible but are less common and are less likely to present with diffuse pulmonary infiltrates.

Tuberculosis could certainly cause both this patient's pulmonary and central nervous system (CNS) problems. The absence of pulmonary adenopathy in a person with advanced AIDS and tuberculosis is not uncommon. The chest CT pattern could be consistent with TB. However, the CSF formula is unusual for tuberculous meningitis, which usually has a protein value higher than 100 and a very low glucose level.

Syphilis can cause a variety of CNS syndromes, including stroke, but this patient's EIA was negative, and syphilis is not an explanation for his pulmonary syndrome.

The suggestion of basal ganglia infarcts on the admitting head CT was provocative. Although ventriculitis can be seen in a number of conditions, including TB and syphilis, it is a hallmark of cytomegalovirus (CMV) CNS infections. An early ophthalmologic examination disclosed that the patient had bilateral CMV retinitis. Subsequently, CMV DNA was found by PCR in the CSF, which was negative for JC virus, BK virus (BKV), herpes simplex virus (HSV), and varicella zoster virus (VZV). At bronchoscopy, a transbronchial biopsy was obtained, which was strongly positive for CMV proteins on immunostaining and negative for other pathogens, including *Pneumocystis*.

TREATMENT

This patient had an overwhelming CMV infection, which was documented to involve his eyes, brain, and lungs—and likely also involved his gut as the cause of his diarrhea. The question is whether this patient warrants treatment with more than one agent.

The evolution of resistance is driven by several factors, including the inherent degree of mutability of the organism and size of the replicating population. HIV has an extremely high rate of mutation and requires treatment with multiple agents simultaneously. The herpesviruses have relatively low intrinsic rates of mutation due to their large and complex genomes, which are intolerant of errors. However, when the population of replicating virus is large, the chance of selecting for resistance is very high. For example, this evolutionary principle underlies the need for multiple agents to treat active TB, while isoniazid or rifampin alone suffices for latent TB. It is also to be found in the treatment of various cancers and leukemias.

In CMV therapy, there is direct evidence for the superiority of combination therapy in the Studies of the Ocular Complications of AIDS (SOCA) study of relapsed CMV retinitis in AIDS in a randomized trial, as well as in retrospective reviews of CMV encephalitis. In these studies, the combination of ganciclovir and foscarnet outperformed single-drug treatment or historical controls.

This patient received 3 weeks of a combination of ganciclovir and foscarnet with resolution of his pulmonary infiltrates, normalization of his pulse oximetry, and resolution of his diarrhea and retinal disease. His degree of alertness improved somewhat, but he remained severely incapacitated by his multiple strokes.

KEY POINTS TO REMEMBER

- Ventriculitis is a hallmark of CMV encephalitis.
- A retinal examination may be very helpful in elucidating a pathogen in patients living with AIDS with CNS disease.
- Tree-in-bud opacities are a radiologic appearance, not a microbiologic diagnosis; many things can cause it.
- In severe CMV disease, especially involving the CNS, combination therapy is recommended.

Further Reading

Anduze-Faris BM, Fillet A-M, Gozlan J, et al. Induction and maintenance therapy of cytomegalovirus central nervous system infection in HIV-infected patients. *AIDS.* 2000;14(5):517–524.

Arribas JR, Storch GA, Clifford DB, Tselis AC. Cytomegalovirus encephalitis. *Ann Intern Med.* 1996;125(7):577–587.

Combination foscarnet and ganciclovir therapy versus monotherapy for the treatment of relapsed cytomegalovirus retinitis in patients with AIDS. The Cytomegalovirus Retreatment Trial. *Arch Ophthalmol* 1996;114(1):23–33.

12 "I've been rashed and confused": Part 2

David E. Barker

A 45-year-old man presents with his third recurrence of herpes zoster involving the left posterior chest. The patient states that the first episode occurred 1 year ago and resolved promptly with oral acyclovir treatment. A second episode occurred 7 months later in the same area and resolved much more slowly on valacyclovir. The patient states currently that despite valacyclovir prophylaxis he has developed a third episode that has been present for the past 4 days in the same area of the chest. He denies fever or systemic symptoms and claims he is compliant with his valacylcovir and HIV medications. A recent CD4 count was 320, and his viral load has been undetectable for several years on combination antiretroviral therapy.

The patient is afebrile, and all vital signs are normal. Examination of the skin of the chest reveals clusters of small vesicles over the posterior and lateral chest in areas with scarring from prior episodes. The lesions appear to cross into adjacent dermatomes and are not perfectly aligned with the course of the ribs above and below the involved area.

What Do You Do Now?

HERPES GLADIATORUM

The presentation suggests that all is not right with the diagnosis of herpes zoster. First, although persons living with HIV (PLWH) have a much higher incidence of recurrent herpes zoster (20%–30%) rather than persons not living with HIV-uninfected persons (5%–8%), the chance of having a second episode within 1 year in a PLWH is about 10%. The next telltale hint is that this disease keeps recurring in the same area. When a second occurrence of zoster does crop up, it is often in a different area. Recurrences of all herpesviruses are due to weakened cell-mediated immunity, as occurs in PLWH. However, varicella zoster virus (VZV) is acquired through an airborne route, causes viremia, and infects all the sensory neurons throughout the body, while herpes simplex virus (HSV), acquired directly through the skin or mucosa, generally only affects the locale into which was inoculated. The repeated recurrence in the same area is an atypical behavior for VZV. Last, VZV recurs in a dermatomal fashion, and although it may spread to adjacent dermatomes or may disseminate and cause widely distributed lesions, the presence of lesions in part of one skin dermatome and part of another adjacent dermatome without ever involving the rest of that dermatome strains understanding.

The alternative condition that is much more likely to recur repeatedly, which mimics the appearance of zoster lesions and is caused by direct inoculation—so it may indeed ignore dermatomal distributions—is herpes gladiatorum. It is named for direct inoculation of the skin during a wrestling match, where virus from herpes oralis is inoculated into a trivial scrape on an opponent's skin. HSV is much more likely to recur multiple times within a year, especially the first year after acquisition. A sample of cells from the base of an unroofed lesion is submitted for immunofluorescence and is positive for HSV antigens and negative for VZV proteins.

Because of the recurrence while on valacyclovir and the history of slow resolution previously, a sample is submitted for culture and sensitivity testing. Sequencing of the virus grown in culture demonstrates a missense mutation in the HSV thymidine kinase gene, which confers resistance to acyclovir and valacyclovir.

TREATMENT

Because the patient's lesions progressed despite high-dose oral valacyclovir, he was admitted and received intravenous foscarnet with good response and resolution after 9 days. Foscarnet is an analogue of pyrophosphate and competes with all the nucleotide triphosphates in the active site of the viral polymerase; it does not require activation by a viral enzyme. Options for oral prophylaxis are limited in a patient with acyclovir-resistant virus, and valacyclovir should be discontinued. Future recurrences may consist of resistant virus, sensitive virus, or mixtures of both.

KEY POINTS TO REMEMBER

- Zoster does not recur as frequently as herpes.
- When zoster recurrences do occur, they are likely to not be in the same dermatome.
- Herpes gladiatorum often mimics zoster lesions but may ignore dermatomes, depending on how it was inoculated into the skin.
- Herpes simplex is more likely to develop resistance to nucleoside antivirals.

Further Reading

Goodman, JL, Holland, EJ, Andres, CW, et al. Epidemiologic notes and reports herpes gladiatorum at a high school wrestling camp—Minnesota. *MMWR Morb Mortal Wkly Rep.* 1990;39(5):69–71.

Levin MJ, Bacon TH Leary JJ. Resistance of herpes simplex virus infections to nucleoside analogues in HIV-infected patients. *Clin Infect Dis.* 2004;39(suppl 5):S248–S257.

Safrin S, Crumpacker C, Chatis P. A controlled trial comparing foscarnet with vidarabine for acyclovir-resistant mucocutaneous herpes simplex in the acquired immunodeficiency syndrome. *N Engl J Med.* 1992;325:551–555.

13 "I've been rashed and confused": Part 3

David E. Barker

A 41-year-old man presents with acute onset of confusion. He was diagnosed with HIV many years ago, with an initial CD4 count of 180. Since that time, he has been on antiretroviral therapy with virologic suppression, and his most recent CD4 count was 480. Other than HIV he has no risk factors for atherosclerosis. Past history includes a mild case of right trigeminal herpes zoster 4 months previously, which resolved rapidly with valacyclovir.

Upon exam he is healthy-appearing with normal vital signs, and entirely unremarkable except for his neurological findings. He has focal weakness in the left upper extremity involving the triceps 3–4/5. His coordination of movement of the left hand and forearm are diminished. He has some inattention to objects in the left visual field in both eyes. Retinal examination is normal.

Acontrast-enhanced magnetic resonance imaging (MRI) is performed, which reveals five small, discrete acute infarcts involving the right side of the brain, including a portion of the motor cortex, the basal ganglia, and visual cortical areas of the occipital lobe at the gray/white matter junctions. A carotid ultrasound is normal.

What Do You Do Now?

VARICELLA ZOSTER VIRUS VASCULOPATHY

The first question is whether this patient has a typical ischemic stroke and should receive antithrombotic treatment. The answer is probably not. The presence of multiple small ischemic areas located in deep brain areas at the ends of blood vessels' territories suggests that this is a watershed stroke syndrome (10% of all strokes), and the presence of multiple infarcts suggests that the cause is embolic.

A transesophageal echocardiogram is performed; no valvular abnormalities and no intracardiac clots are found. Three sets of blood cultures obtained 6 hours apart from each other before antibiotics were given all remained negative. Serologic testing for *Coxiella*, *Bartonella*, and *Brucella* is all negative. Cardiac monitoring demonstrates only normal sinus rhythm.

Dual antiplatelet therapy is initiated, and a computed tomographic (CT) angiogram of the brain is obtained. CT redemonstrates the small infarcts seen on MRI, but there is no occlusion of any large or medium-size vessel and no abnormal vascular calcifications. There is a questionable anatomic abnormality of the right carotid siphon, resulting in increased diameter of the vessel.

A lumbar puncture is obtained, which reveals a normal opening pressure and normal cell counts and cerebrospinal fluid (CSF) chemistries. Serum syphilis enzyme immunoassay is negative, as is a CSF Venereal Disease Research Laboratory (VDRL) test. Serum and CSF cryptococcal antigen studies are negative. Bacterial and fungal studies are negative. Polymerase chain reaction (PCR) studies of the CSF are negative for JC virus, BK virus (BKV), Epstein-Barr virus (EBV), and herpes simplex virus (HSV), but are positive for varicella zoster virus (VZV).

TREATMENT

Therapy with intravenous acyclovir at 12.5 mg/kg every 8 hours is initiated. Despite treatment, the patient develops additional deficits involving the left upper extremity and new deficits involving the left lower extremity. Repeat MRI scanning discloses no change in the initial infarcts, but several new areas of acute infarction are seen. Foscarnet is added to continuing acyclovir treatment as well as prednisone in a dose of 1 mg/kg per day.

After 10 days of treatment, the patient acutely deteriorates with signs of increased intracranial pressure, and he expired.

At autopsy, the right carotid bulb was found to have an area of thinning of the vessel wall with infiltration of mononuclear and multinucleated inflammatory cells. This necrotic area extended to foci of disruption of the endothelium of the vessel and caused a rupture of the external wall of the artery, resulting in a massive intracranial hemorrhage. VZV antigens could not be found by immunostaining, but on electron microscopy, alphaherpesvirus capsids were found in multiple sections of the damaged vessel.

Varicella zoster virus is capable of many problems due to its unique ability to affect the walls of blood vessels. Zoster is associated with a substantial increase in the risk of stroke and transient ischemic attack, as well as extracranial giant cell arteritis (GCA), ischemic retinitis, transverse myelitis, and aneurysm formation. Stroke syndromes are especially likely to follow zoster ophthalmicus, and it is worth noting that the trigeminal ganglion is directly adjacent to the carotid siphon and provides sensory innervation to the blood vessel. Seventy percent of patients with zoster vasculopathy have a history of cutaneous zoster in the past year, with most cases in the past 4 months. VZV can cause severe necrotizing retinitis, referred to as progressive outer retinal necrosis (PORN), which has some distinguishing features from acute retinal necrosis (ARN), which is usually due to HSV. There may be some overlap in the appearance of ARN and PORN, and examination by an ophthalmologist familiar with PORN should be sought. PORN tends to be much more aggressive than ARN and is much more likely to be bilateral. PCR of a sample of the vitreous fluid from an affected eye (0.1 mL) is usually positive in PORN. Combination therapy with acyclovir and foscarnet is superior to acyclovir alone in PORN and is recommended, although there are no randomized trials of this rather rare condition. Oral antivirals do not achieve sufficient levels in the eye to prevent PORN, and there are many case reports of PORN occurring in patients who were on acyclovir or valacyclovir.

In VZV vasculopathy, there is much more inflammation and less viral replication. Steroids are helpful in GCA, a rheumatological disorder now suspected of being caused by VZV, and most experts recommend them in VZV CNS vasculopathy.

- VZV vasculopathy is common in nonimmunosuppressed hosts and is increased in PLWH. It causes ischemic, hemorrhagic, and aneurysmal stroke.
- Stroke risk is highest in the first month following zoster, common out to 4 months, and remains elevated for at least 1 year.
- Patients who have zoster ophthalmicus are at particularly high risk.
- Prophylactic oral antiviral drugs do not appear to affect the reoccurrence of zoster (and do not prevent VZV-PORN).
- In the absence of encephalitis, CSF may be bland. Anti-VZV CSF immunoglobulin G to serum immunoglobulin G is the most sensitive test. CSF PCR is more rapid and is specific.
- Angiography may reveal mild stenosis with aneurysm dilation. In this case, multiple watershed strokes in the distribution of the middle and posterior cerebral arteries on one side are implicated in an arterial process.

Further Reading

Jansen K, Haastert B, Michalik C, et al. Incidence and risk factors of herpes zoster among HIV-positive patients in the German competence network for HIV/AIDS (KompNet): a cohort study analysis. *BMC Infect Dis.* 2013;*13*: article number 372.

Nagel MA, Jones D, Wyborny A. Varicella zoster virus vasculopathy: the expanding clinical spectrum and pathogenesis. *J Neuroimmunol.* 2017;308:112–117.

14 "Doc, I think I have a hemorrhoid"

Hillary Dunlevy

A 47-year-old male with history of HIV, neuropathy, and seizures presents to discuss an area around his anus. It is occasionally firm, tender, bleeds with wiping after a bowel movement, and has been growing in size for the past year. He is concerned that this is a hemorrhoid but has not treated it. He denies a history of condyloma and has never had an anal Papanicolaou (Pap) test. He reports constipation and uses opiates for chronic pain. He was diagnosed with HIV in 1994, with nadir CD4 of 110 cells/μL. His current CD4 is 300 cells/μL, and HIV-1 RNA is less than 20 copies/μL on emtricitabine, tenofovir alafenamide, darunavir, and cobicistat. He is not sexually active but does have a history of insertive and receptive anal sex with men. He has a 20 pack-year history and smokes a half pack of cigarettes daily. Examination reveals an 8-mm, erythematous, indurated nodule on the right lateral aspect of the perianus.

What Do You Do Now?

ANAL HIGH-GRADE SQUAMOUS INTRAEPITHELIAL LESION

A complaint of a perianal lesion should be directly examined. The differential is broad, and direct examination may improve the clinician's understanding of the pathology of a perianal lesion. The differential includes human papilloma virus (HPV) etiologies, including anal condyloma, anal high-grade squamous intraepithelial lesion (HSIL) and anal squamous cell cancer (SCC). Additional considerations include anal fistula or abscess, anal fissure, herpes simplex virus (HSV), syphilis, anal polyp, skin tag, and hemorrhoid. The patient denies recent sexual activity, making a new sexually transmitted infection less likely. He has a significant history of smoking, which can increase the risk of HPV persistence and anal dysplasia due to HPV. He endorses constipation, which can be associated with skin tags or hemorrhoids. While the symptoms of itching, bleeding, and pain can correlate with many etiologies on the differential, the description of the lesion is most consistent with an HPV-related abnormality. A condyloma is typically soft and rubbery, not a palpable nodule as is described here. Further evaluation with high-resolution anoscopy (HRA), which includes application of 5% acetic acid and evaluation with a colposcope, can be performed to assess the characteristics of the lesion. Lesions related to HPV will appear acetowhite on application of acetic acid, and this patient did have such a lesion. A biopsy must be performed in this case to determine the degree of dysplasia, low-grade squamous intraepithelial lesion (LSIL), HSIL, or anal SCC. In this case, the biopsy demonstrated HSIL.

Anogenital HPV infection is acquired primarily through sexual intercourse, though can be transmitted through other means of physical contact. HPV is linked to almost all cervical cancer and 88% of anal cancers, with HPV 16 the largest contributing genotype. Other types of high-risk HPV that lead to HSIL and can progress to anogenital and oropharyngeal cancers include HPV 18, 31, 33, 35, 39, 45, 51, 52, 56, 58, and possibly 68. HPV can be attributed to 4.5% of cancers around the world or 630,000 cases of HPV-related cancer per year. Cervical cancer accounts for 83% of these cancers, with oropharyngeal, anal, penile, vaginal, and vulvar cancer contributing to the remainder.

It is well established that people living with HIV have higher rates of HPV infection, precancerous changes, and both anal and cervical malignancies.

HPV persistence can lead to anogenital cancer over time. Studies demonstrate mixed results on whether antiretroviral therapy reduces the risk of persistent HPV infection, precancerous lesions, or malignancies. Women with cervical and vulvar abnormalities due to HPV have a higher risk of anal cancer. Cervical cancer rates have decreased in the United States due to recommendations for regular screening for precursors to cervical cancer. Worldwide, cervical cancer is still the leading contributor to HPV-related malignancy. Anal cancer rates in people living with HIV are much higher than that of the general population. The North American AIDS Cohort Collaboration on Research and Design (NA-ACCORD) shows higher rates of anal cancer for people living with HIV. Per 100,000 person-years, rates of anal cancer in men who have sex with men (MSM) are 131, are 46 for other men living with HIV, and are 30 for women living with HIV. These rates are much higher than 1.9 per 100,000 person-years for the general population. There are expected to be 13,170 cases (4250 deaths) of cervical cancer and 8300 new cases (1280 deaths) of anal cancer. The median age of diagnosis for cervical cancer is 50 years and for anal cancer is 62 years. The percentage of individuals surviving to 5 years is similar for cervical and anal cancer, 65.8% and 68.3%, respectively. HPV also leads to 70% of oropharyngeal cancer in the United States, but there is currently no recommendation for screening.

Guidelines for cervical cancer screening in people living with HIV recommend a cervical Pap testing on initiation of HIV care, within 1 year of sexual activity, and no later than 21 years of age. Cervical Pap testing should be repeated at 6–12 months, then annually for 3 years, and if no abnormalities are noted, this is followed by transition to a Pap test every 3 years. For women younger than 30, HPV co-testing is not recommended. For these women, any abnormality should be followed up with colposcopy and directed biopsy with possible treatment. The one exception to this is for atypical cells of undetermined significance (ASCUS), for which repeat Pap testing is done at 6–12 months. For women 30 years or older, co-testing with HPV can be performed at the time of diagnosis and repeated in 3 years if normal. Abnormal cytology should be evaluated by colposcopy, including ASCUS if HPV testing is positive. If HPV testing is positive but cytology is negative, repeat testing is done at a year, followed by colposcopy with any abnormality.

Some guidelines support anal Pap testing and HRA with biopsy. There are no national guidelines for treatment of anal HSIL. The HIV Medicine Association and the New York State Health Department support annual anal Pap testing in people living with HIV with a history of receptive anal intercourse, abnormal cervical Pap test, anogenital condyloma with abnormal Pap test (ASCUS, LSIL, and HSIL) followed with HRA with biopsy. Other organizations, such as the Centers for Disease Control and Prevention and Guidelines for the Prevention and Treatment for Opportunistic Infections, suggest that there is not yet enough evidence to support anal dysplasia screening in people living with HIV.

Human papilloma virus can be prevented through HPV vaccination and condom use. Condom use decreases HPV transmission by 70%. The HPV 9-valent vaccine has been shown to be effective in cervical cancer reduction as well as acquisition of new types of HPV infection and HPV-associated disease. This virus-like particle vaccine for HPV has protection against 9 genotypes of HPV, 2 that cause condyloma (6 and 11) and 7 that are oncogenic (16, 18, 31, 33, 45, 52, and 58). The Advisory Committee on Immunization Practices (ACIP) has routinely recommended HPV vaccination for youth ages 11 to 12 in a 2-dose series (0 and 6–12 months) for those younger than 15 years and a 3-dose series for those 15 years and older (0, 1–2 months, and 6 months). As of 2019, catch-up vaccination is recommended for everyone through age 26, as well as catch-up vaccination for some individuals at risk for new HPV exposure and infection, 27–45 years old. They recommend shared clinical decision-making between a patient and provider to determine if HPV vaccination could be beneficial. Further exposure to new strains of HPV through ongoing sexual activity in a group at high risk for HPV infection and disease, such as people living with HIV, can be considered an indication to vaccinate for HPV. The HPV vaccine has been shown to be highly immunogenic in youth and in a 9-valent HPV immunogenicity trial, the geometric mean antibody titers to high-risk HPV types were non-inferior in women ages 27–45 compared to those 16–26 years of age, hence the expanded age indication. Worldwide distribution of the HPV vaccine has been challenging due to refrigeration requirements and expense.

Studies that have evaluated the effectiveness of HPV vaccination to reduce recurrence of previously occurring HPV-related lesions have not been shown to be clearly effective in people living with HIV. At this time, there is no prospective data that demonstrate the HPV vaccine prevents recurrence of HPV-related dysplasia, though there is ongoing research. Some retrospective analyses of individuals not infected with HIV demonstrated reduction in dysplasia recurrence. These studies looked at surgical removal of cervical dysplasia with or without the HPV vaccine and demonstrated some reduction in recurrence of HSIL lesions in those receiving the vaccine. A prospective study in individuals living with HIV did not demonstrate a clear benefit to reduction in recurrence of anal dysplasia, though suggested a possible benefit to recurrence of oropharyngeal HPV infection.

Nononcogenic strains of HPV that lead to oral and anogenital infections include genotypes 6 and 11, contributing to 90% of anogenital condyloma. These genotypes are covered with the HPV vaccine, which has been shown to decrease the incidence of anogenital condyloma. Condyloma are often uncomfortable due to pruritis and bleeding, although they are not generally painful. There are multiple treatment options for anogenital condyloma, including cryotherapy, podophyllin, trichloroacetic acid (TCA), electrosurgery, sinecatechins, and imiquimod.

Topical treatments used for condyloma include imiquimod and sinecatechins ointment. The 5% imiquimod is applied 3 times nightly per week for up to 16 weeks, with instructions to wash off the cream after 8 hours. Sinecatechins ointment is a green tea extract that can be used for topical treatment of condyloma; the precise action is not known but is thought to inhibit inflammatory cells. This ointment is applied 3 times daily to warts for up to 4 months. Rates of condyloma clearance are up to 58%. Side effects include itching, burning, and pain. TCA can be used on small condyloma with the side effect of burning pain and some recurrence. Cryotherapy involves liquid nitrogen spray to freeze condyloma, which can be mildly painful with blistering of the frozen tissue in the days following. Condyloma can recur, requiring multiple treatments, similar to TCA. Electrosurgery uses high-frequency electric current to coagulate or cauterize abnormal tissue. This treatment is effective, with 94% clearance, but there is recurrence. This procedure requires local anesthesia and can be more painful than other modalities on recovery. Carbon dioxide laser therapy uses heat to remove the abnormal tissue. Both electrosurgery and carbon dioxide lasers can have HPV DNA in the smoke produced, removed with vacuum evacuation.

Women living with HIV receive a cervical Pap test every 1–3 years, and some recommendations for people living with HIV suggest anal dysplasia should be evaluated with an annual anal Pap test in both men and women. An anal Pap test is a collection of cells in the anal canal with a polyester or Dacron swab. Though not typically done, HPV testing can be performed for oncogenic types of HPV. Per recommendations, if abnormal cytology is observed, this is followed by HRA. HRA uses an anoscope inserted 5 cm in the anal canal to view with magnification through a colposcope. Vinegar is applied to the anal mucosa along with Lugol's iodine to demonstrate HPV-associated lesions. Small biopsies are performed without local anesthesia. Perianal lesions that are to be biopsied are injected with local anesthesia due to the change in innervation distal to the dentate line. If biopsy shows HSIL, anal intraepithelial lesions grade 2 or 3, the patient returns for removal. Multiple modalities have been used, including infrared coagulation, carbon dioxide laser, and electrosurgery. Creams, including 5-fluorouracil, cidofovir, and imiquimod, have also been used on lesions. A randomized trial comparing infrared coagulation treatment of HSIL to monitoring over the course of a year showed 62% clearance in the treatment group compared to only 30% in the monitoring group. There are high rates of recurrence of HSIL, and multiple treatments may be required for clearance of HPV-associated lesions.

There is no clear consensus on anal cancer screening, although with increased rates of anal cancer in people living with HIV, there is agreement in the minimum recommendations for annual digital anorectal examination and visual inspection of the anogenital area. A current large, multicenter prospective randomized trial is being conducted to determine if treatment of HSIL leads to reduction in cancer. The Anal Cancer HSIL Outcomes Research (ANCHOR) study aims to enroll over 5000 individuals living with HIV with anal HSIL. This study randomizes individuals 1:1 to either treatment or active monitoring of HSIL lesions and follows participants for 5–8 years. The outcomes of this study will likely lead to the development of national guidelines on anal cancer screening and prevention.

Human papilloma virus leads to 70% of the oropharyngeal cancer in the United States and includes involvement of the base of the tongue and tonsils as well as other areas in the oropharynx. HPV 16 is the most common genotype contributing to cancer. One study projected that there will be more cases of HPV-related oropharyngeal cancer than cervical cancer in 2020. Evaluation of oropharyngeal dysplasia and cancer is limited due to lack of approved and effective diagnostic techniques. Evaluation of HPV infection is performed through oral rinse for HPV DNA, though current use is in research and not available clinically. Unlike cervical and anal dysplasia, there is no standard test to assess for oropharyngeal dysplasia from HPV in the oropharynx. Dysplastic lesions may not be readily visible on direct examination, although areas of oropharyngeal leukoplakia and erythroplakia can indicate dysplasia.

Similar to prevention of anogenital HPV infection and subsequent cancer, there is evidence that HPV vaccination prevents oropharyngeal HPV infection. With vaccination of at least one dose of HPV 6, 11, 16, and 18, the prevalence of infection of these genotypes was 0.11% compared to 1.61% in unvaccinated participants, an 88.2% reduction. Given that the majority of oropharyngeal cancers are associated with HPV, the hope is that there would be a decrease in malignancies as well. Evaluating the effect of vaccination on rates of oropharyngeal cancer is complicated due to the long duration of follow-up and large sample size required to detect a decrease in cancer rates for vaccinated individuals and more studies are needed.

KEY POINTS TO REMEMBER

- People living with HIV have high rates of HPV infection and HPV-related precancerous and malignant lesions.
- The HPV 9-valent vaccine is effective at preventing HPV infection and subsequent HPV-related precancerous and malignant lesions.
- The HPV vaccine is recommended for all individuals starting at age 11 up to age 26 and is recommended for some populations up to age 45 years.
- Guidelines recommend screening for cervical cancer every 1–3 years in people living with HIV, depending on findings.

- There are no definitive guidelines for people for anal cancer screening in people living with HIV, although some organizations support annual anal Pap test followed by HRA for evaluation.
- A multisite, randomized trial is currently enrolling individuals with HIV to determine the role of treatment in anal dysplasia.

Further Reading

de Martel C, Plummer M, Vignat J, Franceschi S. Worldwide burden of cancer attributable to HPV by site, country and HPV type. *Int J Cancer.* 2017;141(4):664–670.

Goldstone SE, Lensing SY, Stier EA, et al. A randomized clinical trial of infrared coagulation ablation versus active monitoring of intra-anal high-grade dysplasia in adults with human immunodeficiency virus infection: an AIDS Malignancy Consortium Trial. *Clin Infect Dis.* 2019;68(7):1204–1212.

Meites E, Szilagyi PG, Chesson HW, Unger ER, Romero JR, Markowitz LE. Human papillomavirus vaccination for adults: updated recommendations of the Advisory Committee on Immunization Practices. *MMWR Morb Mortal Wkly Rep.* 2019;68(32):698–702.

Silverberg MJ, Lau B, Justice AC, et al. Risk of anal cancer in HIV-infected and HIV-uninfected individuals in North America. *Clin Infect Dis.* 2012;54(7):1026–1034.

Wang CC, Palefsky JM. Human papillomavirus related oropharyngeal cancer in the HIV-infected population. *Oral Dis.* 2016;22(suppl I):98–106.

Wang CJ, Palefsky JM. Human papillomavirus (HPV) infections and the importance of HPV vaccination. *Curr Epidemiol Rep.* 2015;2(2):101–109.

Yanofsky VR, Patel RV, Goldenberg G. Genital warts: a comprehensive review. *J Clin Aesthet Dermatol.* 2012;5(6):25–36.

15 "This lump under my jaw doesn't hurt but keeps getting bigger"

Estefania Gauto-Mariotti and
Paul G. Rubinstein

A 49-year-old female presents to the emergency room with growing neck lymphadenopathy, night sweats, and a subjective 30-pound weight loss over 1 month. The patient was diagnosed with HIV 6 years earlier and was noncompliant with her HIV medications. She was taking elvitegravir/cobicistat/emtricitabine/tenofovir disoproxil fumarate. She had extensive lymphadenopathy on imaging, and a biopsy of her neck lymph node and of her bone marrow showed involvement by diffuse large B-cell lymphoma. Initial laboratory tests demonstrated an HIV-1 viral load greater than 1,000,000 copies/mL, and her CD4+ T-cell count is 70 cells/μL. Hepatitis B and C serologies are negative. Other pertinent laboratory findings show a lactate dehydrogenase (LDH) value of 800, a normal liver function test, and normal cardiac ejection fraction.

What Do You Do Now?

NON-HODGKIN AND HODGKIN LYMPHOMA IN PATIENTS LIVING WITH HIV/AIDS

Prior to the implementation of combined antiretroviral therapy (ART) in the mid-1990s, it was clear that the most common cancers affecting people living with HIV/AIDS (PLWHA) were Kaposi sarcoma (KS) and aggressive non-Hodgkin lymphoma. In 1982, the Centers for Disease Control and Prevention determined that a CD4+ T-cell count below 200 cells/μL was insufficient to define AIDS and expanded the definition to all patients diagnosed with primary central nervous system (CNS) lymphoma (PCNSL) and KS. Aggressive non-Hodgkin lymphoma or AIDS-related lymphoma (ARL) and later invasive cervical cancer were also added to the list of "AIDS-defining" cancers (ADCs). These ARLs include PCNSL, Burkitt lymphoma (BL), diffuse large B-cell lymphoma (DLBCL), plasmablastic lymphoma (PL), and primary effusion lymphoma (PEL). As described further in this chapter, prior to ART the median survival was only 8 months for DLBCL. After the initiation of ART, survival improved for ARL. However, it remains one of the leading causes of death currently and carries a large morbidity burden in the HIV-infected population. The purpose of this chapter, in addition to describing the epidemiology, presentation, and outcomes of lymphomas in PLWHA, is an attempt to describe the many aspects in the management of lymphoma unique to this population, including infection prophylaxis during chemotherapy and management of ART/chemotherapy interactions, issues that both the primary HIV physician and an oncologist should be made aware.

Management: Important issues to take into consideration are discussed in this paragraph. (1) Regarding ART know that cobicistat is a strong CYP 3A4 inhibitor that interacts with vincristine. In general, a change to an anti-HIV regimen that has no CYP 3A4 inhibition is done 1 week prior to the initiation of chemotherapy; the ART chosen was efavirez/emtricitabine/tenofovir. The patient was treated with dose-adjusted rituximab, etoposide, prednisone, vincristine, cyclophosphamide, and doxorubicin (daREPOCH). (2) Concerning prophylaxis, the patient was already taking Bactrim for *Pneumocystis jirovecii* pneumonia (PJP) prophylaxis. Azithromycin was added, understanding that with chemotherapy, the CD4+ T-cell count would decrease below 50 cells/μL. Levofloxacin and myeloid growth factor were given for 7–10 days postchemotherapy, every cycle, until neutrophil recovery. The patient was found to have no lymphadenopathy by cycle 3 and was positron emission tomographic (PET) negative after cycle 6. The issues in management in this case are emphasized and discussed in more detail next.

EPIDEMIOLOGY

Since the advent of ART, the prevalence of PLWHA in North America has continued to rise over time, from 800,000 in the year 2000 to 1.17 million in 2018. This was due in large part to the improved survival imparted by ART and the relative constant rate of infection. Recently, the infection rate of HIV has dropped; however, over 1 million people are expected to be infected with HIV/AIDS by the year 2030. Since the implementation of ART, the incidence of ADC has declined. In 1993, over 7000 patients were diagnosed with ARLs in the United States compared to just about 2000 in 2005 despite the increased prevalence. However, in the year 2010, ARLs remained the leading cancer diagnosed and are expected to be the third leading cancer diagnosis in 2020 in PLWHA. Currently, DLBCL is the most common ARL followed by BL. PCNSL and PEL are rarer and normally present in the late stages of HIV (Table 15.1). Retrospective data demonstrated that ADCs represent 7%–15%, and non-AIDS–defining malignancies represent 12%–27% of all deaths in PLWHA, making cancer a leading cause of death. Currently, PLWHA have an 8-fold increased risk of developing HIV-associated classical Hodgkin lymphoma (HIV-cHL) and 12-fold increase risk of developing ARLs over the general population. Even in patients treated with ART, ARLs impart a hazard ratio of death close to 10 compared to the general population.

Classification and Outcomes of Hodgkin and Non-Hodgkin Lymphoma in PLWHA

The definition of ARLs is as aggressive non-Hodgkin lymphomas (Table 15.1). All lymphomas not meeting this definition are non–AIDS defining (e.g., HIV-cHL). The presentation, outcomes, and molecular basis of disease are varied among all of the different ARLs. While the cause of lymphoma is multifactorial, the largest risk factor is a suppressed CD4+ T-cell count. For

TABLE 15.1 **World Health Organization Classification of Lymphomas Associated With HIV Infection**

Burkitt lymphoma	Presents with elevated CD4+ T-cell counts, second most common ARL
Diffuse large B-cell lymphoma (DLBCL)	Most common ARL; usually presents with extranodal disease, most common sites are the CNS "primary CNS lymphoma" (PCNSL), gastrointestinal tract, bone marrow, and liver
Primary effusion/body cavity lymphoma (PEL)	Rare, presents in patients in the late stages of HIV; associated 100% with HHV-8; frequently presents in patients with preexisting Kaposi sarcoma
Plasmablastic lymphoma	Rare, accounts for 2% of all HIV-related lymphomas; associated with HHV-8 50% and EBV 50%; extranodal presentation is most frequent, particularly in the oral cavity or jaw
Classic Hodgkin lymphoma	Non–AIDS-defining lymphoma; presents with elevated CD4+ T-cell counts; most common non–AIDS-defining lymphoma
MALT (mucosa-associated lymphoid tissue(=) lymphoma	Non–AIDS-defining lymphoma; rare in PLWHA
Peripheral T-cell lymphoma	Rare

example, in a retrospective analysis, the standard incidence ratio for ARL increased from 35.8 to 145 compared to that of the non-HIV population when the CD4+ T-cell count decreased from 500 to less than 100 cells/mm^3. The suppressed CD4+ T-cell count can increase the risk of infection or reactivation of oncogenic viruses that can promote lymphomagenesis, in particular that of the gamma-herpesvirus family (Epstein-Barr virus [EBV] and/or human herpesvirus 8 [HHV-8]), also known as Kaposi sarcoma herpesvirus). A retrospective study done at Cook County Hospital in Chicago demonstrated the average CD4+ T-cell count at presentation for PCNSL was just 12 cells/µL. Co-infection with EBV is found in 90%–100% of PCNSL, PL, and HIV-cHL. All cases of PEL are infected with HHV-8 and in most cases are infected additionally with EBV. Most lymphomas occurring in PLWHA present with suppressed CD4+ T-cell counts, BL and HIV-cHL are the exception, and currently 25% of patients diagnosed with lymphoma in PLWHA present with CD4+ T-cell counts above 200 cells/µL. Of interest, it is thought that CD4+ T cells, in the microenvironment of the surrounding lymphoma cells, are required for tumor genesis in the case of BL and HIV-cHL.

Treatment outcomes regardless of the histology have remarkably improved in the ART era. Treatment of HIV-cHL, with standard therapy, doxorubicin, bleomycin, vinblastine, and dacarbazine (ABVD) without ART imparted an overall survival (OS) of 48% at 2 years compared to 78% OS at 5 years when ABVD was given in conjunction with anti-HIV therapy for Stage III/IV HIV-cHL, similar to the non-HIV population. Similar improvements were identified in non-Hodgkin lymphoma. In the pre-ART era, for PLWHA diagnosed with DLBCL the median survival was only 8 months. Recent studies from the AIDS Malignancy Consortium (AMC) demonstrated that therapy in conjunction with ART achieved complete remission rates of 70%–80% and an OS of 75% at 1 year for DLBCL, again, similar to the non-HIV population. An important aspect of therapy is continued ART during chemotherapy. A retrospective study of 1000 ARLs demonstrated that treatment in the presence of ART improved rates of remission and OS. Treatment of both Hodgkin and non-Hodgkin lymphoma in the presence of ART is the current standard. The 2 ARL histologies that continue to remain most resistant to therapy are PL and PEL, which impart an OS at 1 year of only 40%–70% depending on the study. Thus, enrollment of patients with ARL onto clinical trials is imperative to continue to improve outcomes. New targeted therapies, daratumumab and brentuximab vedotin, for these lymphomas are currently being studied by the AMC.

While the specific treatment of each malignancy is at the discretion of the treating oncologist, in the ART era, the therapeutic options available to the non-HIV population can be given safely to the HIV population, with similar outcomes if certain principles are maintained (described in the following).

Presentation, Diagnostic Evaluations, and Treatment Principles of Hodgkin and Non-Hodgkin Lymphoma in PLWHA

The clinical presentation of lymphoma in patients with HIV are similar to those seen in the general population (e.g., nontender lymphadenopathy and constitutional B signs/symptoms [10% weight loss, fever, and night sweats]). In addition to a careful history of symptoms, a medication assessment is imperative to avoid potential chemotherapy/ART/concomitant medication interactions. If concerned for malignancy, the patient should be referred to an oncologist. If a biopsy is considered, only core or excisional biopsy should be performed. The diagnostic evaluation should include a complete physical examination focusing on evidence of lymphadenopathy and hepato/splenomegaly. The HHV-8 virus, the cause of KS, is also the oncogenic virus responsible for multicentric Castleman disease (MCD) and PEL. Many cases of PEL and MCD present with concominant KS; thus, a careful skin examination may give a clue regarding the etiology of an effusion or lymphadenopathy. For a patient with KS with a new effusion or new lymphadenopathy, the etiology should be aggressively pursued.

Laboratory evaluation should assess for cytopenias; liver function, including LDH; and hepatitis co-infection. Specific laboratory tests needed in the PLWHA are CD4+ T-cell count and HIV-1 viral load. Imaging studies include a computerized tomographic (CT) scan of the chest, abdomen, and pelvis or a whole-body PET/CT scan.

CONCLUSION

A 12-fold increased risk of being diagnosed with ARL and an 8-fold increase of being diagnosed with HIV-cHL exists for PLWHA over that of the general population. In 2020, ARL is expected to be the third most common diagnosed malignancy in the HIV population. While the morbidity and mortality of ARL are substantial, in the ART era, outcomes of ARL and HIV-cHL have become similar to the non-HIV population. Some lymphoma histologies continue to impart a poor diagnosis, particularly PL and PEL; thus, patients with HIV and lymphoma should be referred for clinical trials if possible so outcomes can continue to improve, particularly in this era of targeted therapy. In the presence of ART, therapies are usually as well tolerated as in the non-HIV population, including that of stem cell transplantation. Careful attention needs to be placed on infection prophylaxis and chemotherapy/ART/concomitant medication interactions, and with a multidiscipline approach, outcomes will be maximized.

There are certain principles of therapy that should be maintained for any cancer patient who has HIV; the ones described apply to both the oncologist and the primary HIV provider.

- Treatment should be given with a multidisciplinary team if possible, including a pharmacist, HIV primary care provider, and an oncologist.
- As a general rule, the CD4+T-cell count drops about 30%–50% with chemotherapy and may take 1 year to recover. Therefore, all patients should receive prophylaxis for PCP regardless of the CD4+T-cell count. Additionally, if the CD4+T-cell count is suspected to drop below 50 cells/μL, prophylaxis for *Mycobacterium avium* should also be initiated, as recommended by the AMC.
- All patients being treated for ARL should receive hematopoietic growth factor, and patients with a CD4+T-cell count below 100 should also receive quinolone prophylaxis, as these patients are at higher risk of infection.
- ART/chemotherapy interactions are a fluid subject as new anti-HIV medications are always being introduced. Many chemotherapeutic agents are cleared through the liver via the CYP 3A4 pathway. The antiretroviral medications with strong CYP 3A4 inhibitory properties, commonly used in HIV therapy (e.g., cobicistat or ritonavir), should be avoided and changed to a noncobicistat or nonritonavir regimen 1 week prior to chemotherapy initiation. Consultation with a pharmacist with expertise in HIV therapy is recommended, and interactions with all medications and chemotherapy should be assessed.
- Hepatitis co-infection with HIV is common in PLWHA. Hepatitis B reactivation has been demonstrated in the non-HIV population

receiving rituximab or immunosuppressive chemotherapy. PLWHA can safely be given chemotherapy with little risk of reactivation if an ART regimen is chosen to cover for hepatitis (e.g., tenofovir).

Further Reading

Noy A. Optimizing treatment of HIV-associated lymphoma. *Blood*. 2019 24;134(17):1385–1394.

Rubinstein PG, Aboulafia DM, Zloza A. Malignancies in HIV/AIDS: from epidemiology to therapeutic challenges. *AIDS*. 2014;28(4):453–465. doi:10.1097/QAD.0000000000000071

Shiels MS, Islam JY, Rosenberg PS, Hall HI, Jacobson E, Engels EA. Projected cancer incidence rates and burden of incident cancer cases of HIV infected adults in the United States through 2030. *Ann Intern Med*. 2018;168:866–873.

16 Sex, Drugs, and Acholic Stools

Sarah A. Rojas and Christian B. Ramers

A 24-year-old man with HIV presents for an unscheduled visit. He complains of several weeks of fatigue, myalgias, nausea, anorexia, and light-colored stools. His friends have told him that his "color has changed," and he thinks his eyes may be turning yellow. He is a regular clinic patient diagnosed with HIV infection 2 years prior. He started antiretroviral therapy (ART) 2 weeks after initial diagnosis, which he has tolerated well. He has no chronic medical problems but has a history of rectal chlamydia and syphilis. He drinks 4–5 alcoholic beverages per night on weekends and has a stimulant use disorder in remission. He has been abstinent for over a year except for a "meth bender" 6 weeks prior. He denies ever injecting drugs. He has sex with men and has one regular partner who is HIV negative; however, 6 weeks ago he participated in a "sex party" with 4 male partners of unknown HIV status. Hepatitis A, B, and C antibody testing was negative at baseline on initial HIV diagnosis, and repeat screening during this visit is also negative.

> **What Do You Do Now?**

ACUTE HEPATITIS C INFECTION

Discussion

The hepatitis C virus (HCV) is typically thought of as a blood-borne pathogen most commonly transmitted through transfusions; nonsterile tattoos; sharing of needles, syringes, or equipment during intravenous drug use; or from mother to child. More recently, outbreaks of sexually transmitted HCV have been reported, initially among men who have sex with men (MSM), particularly those living with HIV and/or using drugs or alcohol during sexual activity. Because of the extremely low observed rates of HCV transmission among sero-discordant heterosexual couples, sexual transmission of HCV is thought to behave differently from a typical sexually transmitted infection and may actually represent microscopic blood exposure rather than transmission through sexual fluids. Because HCV can survive longer when exposed to air outside the body, up to 3 weeks, compared to HIV, for which concentrations in dried blood are very low to negligible, and has been known to be transmitted by sharing razors, toothbrushes, and even straws used for intranasal drugs, many people living with HCV are not able to identify a specific risk factor.

Differential Diagnosis

In patients presenting with an acute icteric illness, liver disease in various forms must be at the top of the differential diagnosis. Toxic liver injury can occur after exposure to herbal supplements, excessive alcohol, acetaminophen, and other more rare exposures (e.g., mushrooms, chemicals, other drugs); however, none of these details is mentioned in this case, and those clinical presentations are typically more acute. Theoretically, any of the hepatitis viruses may cause an acute or subacute hepatitis syndrome; however, in the United States, social and contextual clues can typically narrow the list to hepatitis A, B, or C.

Although vaccination against the hepatitis A virus (HAV) has been universally recommended in the United States as part of the routine childhood immunization series since 2006, many adults remain nonimmune and thus at risk for food-borne or person-to-person transmission. In fact, numerous outbreaks of hepatitis A have been described in recent years associated with homelessness and drug use, likely representing oral-fecal transmission.

Diagnosis of acute HAV is accomplished with antibody testing for anti-HAV immunoglobulin (Ig) M and IgG. Hepatitis B virus (HBV) vaccine has been recommended in the United States for all infants since 1991; however, there remain many adults without protective immunity. Patients immigrating from countries endemic for HBV, particularly in Asia or Africa, may present with an acute HBV flare that may be indistinguishable from other forms of acute viral hepatitis. Diagnostic testing for acute HBV or HBV flare is a bit more difficult but can be made with an HBV surface antigen test, the total and IgM "core" antibody test, and measurement of an HBV DNA viral load. There is no vaccine for hepatitis C, so any exposed patient is at risk.

Clinical Presentation

Acute hepatitis C is defined not by symptoms but also by the estimated time of exposure to disease, with 6 months being the arbitrary cutoff between acute and chronic infection. The rationale for using this time period to distinguish acute from chronic HCV is based on evidence that roughly two-thirds of those who spontaneously clear HCV have done so by 6 months. Only about 15%–25% of patients with acute HCV will exhibit symptoms in the first 4–12 weeks after exposure (mean 7–8 weeks). Fulminant hepatic failure can occur more frequently with HAV and HBV but is extremely rare in acute HCV. Symptoms of acute HCV described in the literature in decreasing frequency are jaundice, flu-like symptoms, dark urine/light stool, nausea, and abdominal pain. Patients with symptomatic acute HCV, particularly with icteric disease, have been observed to have higher rates of spontaneous clearance. All patients with acute hepatitis of any variety will have elevated transaminase levels, typically greater than 5-fold the upper limit of normal and occasionally greater than 1000 IU/mL. Toxic liver injury, acetaminophen overdose, and hepatitis A will generally cause much higher elevations in transaminase levels than acute HCV. Bilirubin levels are almost always elevated, and alkaline phosphatase levels can be variable.

Epidemiology

The Centers for Disease Control and Prevention (CDC) estimated that more than 2 million individuals are living with HCV in the United States. Several specific populations appear to be more affected than others. For example, baby boomers—those born between 1945 and 1965—were noted to have HCV rates of around 3- to 5-fold higher than the general population, probably due to a plurality of exposures. Perhaps most importantly, the blood supply in the United States was not routinely screened until July 1992, and universal precautions demanding personal protective equipment and sterile instruments were not widely implemented until after the HIV/AIDS epidemic took hold in the 1980s. Furthermore, sterile technique and the avoidance of multiuse vials of medicines, vaccines, or other materials such as ink likely were not fully implemented by tattoo parlors and dental and medical offices until the early 1990s. From the early 2000s onward, HCV transmission has largely been fueled by the opioid epidemic, with new infection rates rising every year between 2013 and 2020, particularly in people who inject drugs.

People living with HIV are known to have higher rates of HCV infection than the general population, largely because of shared transmission routes of the two viruses. Early cohorts from North America and Europe reported that up to 25% of people living with HIV also had HCV co-infection. Historically, emphasis was placed on injection drug use to explain HIV/HCV co-infection; however, several outbreaks of sexually transmitted HCV in individuals living with HIV have more recently been described. Because of a widespread effort to engage those with HIV in care, many HIV/HCV co-infected patients have already been identified, treated, and cured of their HCV, so the rate of co-infection is likely to be much lower now. Finally, MSM without HIV, particularly those taking HIV preexposure prophylaxis (PrEP) who have multiple sexual partners are at risk for sexual transmission of HCV, and annual HCV testing is indicated for those taking PrEP.

Diagnostic Testing

In 2019, the CDC, US Preventive Services Task Force, and American Association for the Study of Liver Disease/Infectious Diseases Society of America (AASLD/IDSA) have all revised their guidelines to recommend universal screening for HCV in the general adult population. When screening the general population for HCV, the recommended testing sequence is to start with an HCV antibody test (either a rapid test using a fingerstick or traditional enzyme-linked immunosorbent assay using whole blood). If this is negative, and the patient does not report any recent exposures, then he or she does not have HCV infection. A positive HCV antibody test should prompt the clinician to then send a sample for an HCV RNA test, also known as a "viral load," to see if the infection is currently active. Some laboratories bypass the need for a clinician's order and conduct reflex testing; that is, they may automatically run an HCV RNA test on all positive HCV antibody specimens. By definition, a positive viral load detected more than 6 months following exposure is considered a chronic infection (Figure 16.1). An individual with recent exposure may not have developed HCV antibodies yet and thus might be in the "window period." This is the situation in the clinical vignette, where the exposure was only 6 weeks prior to presentation, so the HCV antibody was still negative. An HCV RNA or viral load examination is the only way to diagnose acute HCV infection in these scenarios.

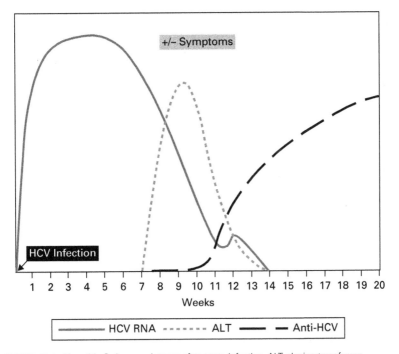

FIGURE 16.1 Hepatitis C virus persistence after acute infection. ALT, alanine transferase. Illustration from David H. Spach, MD.

Treatment and Management Considerations

Guidelines on how to approach acute HCV infection have changed dramatically with the advent of all-oral, well-tolerated, direct-acting antiviral (DAA) regimens, boasting high rates of HCV cure, defined by an "undetectable" HCV RNA or viral load, shown from samples drawn 12 weeks after the completion of therapy, the so-called Sustained Virologic Response (SVR)12. HCV treatment in "interferon era" involved long courses of therapy, weekly injections, and many pills with major side effects and relatively low success rates. Still, it was observed that curing HCV was a bit easier in the acute setting than in the chronic phase, perhaps adding 10%–15% above a relatively low 40%–50% success rate. Clinicians would often debate whether to wait to see if the patient would spontaneously clear (Figure 16.2) the virus or to offer a potentially toxic therapy with a relatively higher chance of cure. The advent of well-tolerated DAA regimens

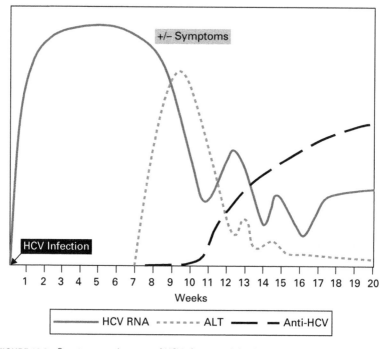

FIGURE 16.2 Spontaneous clearance of HCV after acute infection. Illustration from David H. Spach, MD.

has tipped this dilemma significantly toward treating rather than watchful waiting; however, cost and access considerations continue to complicate decision-making in situations of acute HCV.

In November 2019, the AASLD/IDSA guidelines recommended treating all patients with acute HCV and confirmed viremia rather than waiting several months for spontaneous resolution. Two main reasons for this change were offered: (1) Real-world data and mathematical modeling have shown that immediate treatment will lead to decreases in prevalence and incidence of HCV infection; and (2) a several-month delay in initiation of DAA treatment may be associated with loss to follow-up. In support of the concept of HCV "treatment as prevention," the AIDS Therapy Evaluation in the Netherlands (ATHENA) Dutch cohort of people living with HIV has had a 51% decrease in acute HCV infection after implementation of unrestricted access to DAA-based HCV treatment. Furthermore, investigators in Germany recently observed that if HCV RNA does not dramatically drop (more than 2 log) within 4–6 weeks, 97% of patients will remain chronically infected. On a practical basis, if patients are symptomatic, DAA treatment may be the only action that can alleviate symptoms. And finally, given the World Health Organization's goal to achieve HCV elimination by 2030, the treatment of acute HCV would likely contribute by reducing both prevalence and potentially onward transmission.

A standard workup of a newly diagnosed person with HCV includes a complete history and physical examination (with particular attention to the social history); basic laboratory investigations (complete blood count, metabolic panel); tests for other blood-borne pathogens (HIV, HBV); and a complete abdominal ultrasound. An assessment of the degree of fibrosis must be conducted, preferably with noninvasive methods, such as serological estimates (FibroTest, AST to Platelet Ratio Index [APRI], Fib-4), or elastography, an ultrasound-based tool that can estimate fibrosis by assessing liver stiffness through the intercostal space. Liver biopsy is no longer recommended or required prior to HCV treatment. Testing urine for drugs of abuse or alcohol does not predict treatment adherence and is not required in many areas. It is important, however, to identify secondary liver diseases such as alcoholic hepatitis or cirrhosis and to facilitate addiction treatment for any ongoing substance use disorders identified in the pretreatment workup.

With respect to choice of DAA therapy, there are now many options available, each with greater than 95% cure rates. The AASLD/IDSA guidelines offer a simplified algorithm for uncomplicated cases, in which patients may be treated with a pan-genotypic regimen such as sofosbuvir/velpatasvir for 12 weeks or glecaprevir/pibrentasvir for 8 weeks with minimal clinical or laboratory monitoring. For those with more complex clinical presentations, including HIV co-infection, a careful initial evaluation and follow-up plan should be undertaken.

HIV/HCV co-infection is associated a lower rate of spontaneous clearance and more rapid progression of liver fibrosis and cirrhosis, including some reports of ultrarapid progression from acute infection to cirrhosis within a few years. In contrast, through the many clinical trials of DAA agents, it has been demonstrated that HIV co-infection bears very little impact on the ability to achieve sustained virologic response, or "cure." In fact, if one were to make a cross-study comparison, many HIV/HCV co-infection trials reported higher cure rates than those enrolling HCV mono-infected patients. Currently, one of the only unique considerations particular to the patient with HIV/HCV co-infection is the identification and management of drug-drug interactions between ART regimens and DAAs. In general, regimens based on an integrase strand transfer inhibitor tend to have fewer interactions than non-nucleoside reverse transcriptase inhibitors (NNRTIs) or protease inhibitors (PIs). A thorough investigation using a validated drug-drug interaction database such as the University of Liverpool database (https://www.hep-druginteractions.org) is recommended.

CASE RESOLUTION AND CONCLUSION

Acute HCV has been seen with increasing frequency in young people who inject drugs as well as MSM, particularly those who are living with HIV. Chronicity of infection can be distinguished with HCV antibody and HCV RNA as well as a detailed social history to identify exposures. In the clinical vignette, a sexual exposure 6 weeks prior to presentation, as well as a negative HCV antibody test and positive HCV RNA result confirm that this was an episode of acute hepatitis C. Treatment is now recommended for all with viremic HCV infection, rather than watchful waiting, to engage patients quickly and to decrease the potential for onward transmission. DAA regimens are well tolerated and all oral and yield cure (SVR12) rates of more than 95%, even in HIV/HCV co-infected patients, in as little as 2 to 3 months of treatment. The recommendations for cured patients for: (1) ongoing HCC surveillance if F3 or greater at pre-treatment baseline; (2) post-SVR12 screening with RNA NAAT if risk factors for re-exposure persist. As in any patient with HCV infection, pretreatment staging of liver fibrosis is essential in order to triage the care pathway of patients once they are cured. Those with moderate–to-severe fibrosis (e.g., METAVIR Stage F3 or F4) need ongoing surveillance for hepatocellular carcinoma (HCC). Screening for reinfection with annual HCV RNA testing is recommended for populations with ongoing risk (people who use drugs or MSM) or for any additional known high-risk exposure.

KEY POINTS TO REMEMBER

- Acute HCV can present like other forms of acute hepatitis with jaundice, nausea, fatigue, myalgias, dark urine, and acholic stools.
- Diagnosis of acute HCV requires a positive viral load or HCV RNA test. HCV antibodies usually develop within 1–2 months.
- Transmission of HCV is most efficient through blood exposure from sharing of needles, syringes, or other drug use paraphernalia; however, transmission has been described through sharing razors, toothbrushes, straws to inhale drugs, or sexual exposure, particularly unprotected anal intercourse.
- Roughly 75% of those exposed to HCV will go on to develop a chronic infection, which, if untreated, can cause liver inflammation and lead to cirrhosis, liver cancer, and death.
- Treatments for HCV have improved dramatically with the arrival in 2013 of combination all–oral, direct-acting antivirals (DAAs), which now offer cure rates of more than 95% with just 2 or 3 months of all-oral therapy.

Further Reading

Chan DPC, Sun HY, Wong HTH, Lee SS, Hung CC. Sexually acquired hepatitis C virus infection: a review. *Int J Infect Dis.* 2016;49:47–58. doi:10.1016/j.ijid.2016.05.030

IDSA/AASLD. Management of acute HCV Infection. HCV guidance: recommendations for testing, managing, and treating hepatitis C. https://www.hcvguidelines.org/printpdf/node/666/page-pdf?file=507-UniqueAcute Infection. Published 2018. Accessed January 21, 2020.

Naggie S, Fierer DS, Hughes M, et al. 100% SVR with 8 weeks of ledipasvir/sofosbuvir in HIV-infected men with acute HCV infection: results from the SWIFT-C trial. *Hepatology.* 2017;66(suppl):196.

Nijmeijer BM, Koopsen J, Schinkel J, Prins M, Geijtenbeek TBH. Sexually transmitted hepatitis C virus infections: current trends, and recent advances in understanding the spread in men who have sex with men. *J Int AIDS Soc.* 2019;22(S6):e25348. doi:10.1002/jia2.25348

Rockstroh JK, Lacombe K, Viani RM, et al. Efficacy and safety of glecaprevir/pibrentasvir in patients coinfected with hepatitis C virus and human immunodeficiency virus type 1: the EXPEDITION-2 study. *Clin Infect Dis.* 2018;67(7):1010–1017.

University of Liverpool. HEP interactions. https://www.hep-druginteractions.org/. Accessed January 21, 2020.

US Department of Health and Human Services. Hepatitis C virus infection. Guidelines for the prevention and treatment of opportunistic infections in adults and adolescents with HIV. Published 2019. https://aidsinfo.nih.gov/guidelines/html/4/adult-and-adolescent-opportunistic-infection/345/hepatitis-c-virus. Accessed January 21, 2020.

Wyles D, Bräu N, Kottilil S, et al. Sofosbuvir and velpatasvir for the treatment of hepatitis C virus in patients coinfected with human immunodeficiency virus type 1: an open-label, phase 3 study. *Clin Infect Dis.* 2017; 65(1): 6–12.

17 "I did have some cough when I was still living in Africa six months ago"

L. Beth Gadkowski and Connie Haley

A 45-year-old woman presents to the emergency department complaining of productive cough, dyspnea, weight loss, and fever for 2 weeks. She is a physician and thought she had the flu, but her symptoms have not improved. She currently lives in the United States but is originally from South Africa. She regularly travels back and forth to South Africa for work and to visit family, most recently 6 months ago. Her medical history is significant for malaria and latent tuberculosis (TB) infection (LTBI), for which she received 6 months of isoniazid 15 years ago. On presentation, her temperature is 39°C, respiratory rate is 25, blood pressure is 100/70 mm Hg, heart rate is 110 beats per minute, and O_2 saturation is 91% on room air. She is ill-appearing, with prominent cervical lymphadenopathy and oral thrush. She has rhonchi bilaterally, and breath sounds are decreased in the right lower lobe. A chest x-ray shows scattered reticulonodular infiltrates, hilar lymphadenopathy, and a moderate right pleural effusion. After verbal consent, a rapid HIV returns positive.

What Do You Do Now?

DISCUSSION TB IN HIV INFECTION

The differential diagnosis for a person with untreated HIV, respiratory symptoms, and bilateral infiltrates with hilar adenopathy includes a variety of opportunistic infections and endemic mycoses, as well as malignancy and non–HIV-related conditions. However, this woman's clinical presentation in context of prior LTBI (even if presumably treated, which reduces risk of active TB by 80% if taken) and having emigrated from South Africa, where she worked as a physician make TB a primary diagnostic consideration.

Globally, 10 million persons develop TB each year, and 1 in 4 persons is infected with *Mycobacterium tuberculosis* (*Mtb*) with future risk of TB. Patients with HIV co-infection have substantially increased risk for both acquiring *Mtb* infection and progression from infection to TB disease regardless of CD4 T-cell count. In turn, TB ramps up HIV replication and reduces CD4 cell recovery, hastening progression to AIDS and death. Medical providers are thus encouraged to "think TB" to enable early diagnosis and treatment.

Clinical Presentation and Diagnosis

The initial steps when TB is suspected are to isolate the patient, obtain appropriate diagnostic samples, and notify the local public health department (PHD). If a patient does not otherwise require hospitalization, the patient can be isolated at home if under the supervision of the PHD. For this patient, hospitalization is necessary given her hypoxia and severity of illness. Given her immunosuppression, appropriate diagnostic testing should be obtained quickly to enable appropriate treatment and avoid rapid deterioration.

Tubercular disease most often involves the lungs but can occur at any site throughout the body. In patients with HIV co-infection, TB presentation varies with immune competence. At higher CD4 T-cell counts, TB may manifest with a "classic" presentation, such as fever, night sweats, weight loss, productive cough, and upper lobe infiltrates and/or cavitary lesions on chest x-ray. Subclinical TB can occur with minimal symptoms and even a normal chest radiograph, but microbiologic confirmation of *Mtb*. As immunodeficiency progresses, clinical presentation may be atypical, including noncavitary infiltrates in the middle and lower lung lobes, and extrapulmonary disease becomes more common, such as lymphadenitis, pleuritis, pericarditis, and meningitis. TB may widely disseminate and progress to bacteremia, sepsis, and death if not treated.

HIV providers should maintain a high index of suspicion for TB, particularly among patients with risk of TB exposure, such as birth or residence in TB-endemic areas (most countries in Latin America, the Caribbean, Africa, Asia, Eastern Europe, and Russia); contacts to pulmonary TB; work or residence in high-risk congregate settings (e.g., correctional facilities, homeless shelters, etc.); and healthcare workers who care for patients at high risk for TB. In addition to HIV, risk factors for progression to TB disease after *Mtb* infection include recent infection, low body weight, diabetes, advanced renal disease, malignancy, use of tumor necrosis factor-alpha inhibitors or other immunosuppressive therapies.

Diagnosis of TB should be aggressively pursued rather than initiating empiric therapy without confirmation. A tuberculin skin test (TST) or interferon-gamma release assay (IGRA) would not be an appropriate *initial* test to establish a diagnosis of active TB disease, but may help to increase the suspicions of active TB disease by indicating if the person has been infected with *Mtb*. However, these tests cannot distinguish between LTBI and active TB disease. The sensitivity of these screening tests is decreased in immunocompromised patients, so a negative TST or IGRA *does not rule out active TB disease.*

A posterior-anterior and lateral chest x-ray should always be obtained if clinical findings suggest TB, even in persons without pulmonary symptoms. It is not uncommon for patients living with HIV to present with prominent extrapulmonary complaints and have pulmonary TB detected incidentally. Three or more sputum samples should be collected 8 hours apart with at least 1 early morning specimen. If the patient cannot produce a natural sputum sample, sputum induction should be attempted as it has both a higher yield and favorable cost-analysis compared to bronchoscopy. If bronchoscopy is required, obtain a postbronchoscopy sputum sample, which has yield as high as 80% among patients living with HIV. Appropriate specimens should also be collected from extrapulmonary sites where indicated.

Clinical samples should be sent to the microbiology laboratory for acid-fast bacilli (AFB) smear, mycobacterial culture, and conventional drug susceptibility testing (DST). Because AFB smears are neither specific nor sensitive for *Mtb*, and cultures with growth-based DST take weeks or months to provide results, nucleic acid amplification testing (NAAT) to detect *Mtb* DNA should be performed directly on at least 1 specimen. Molecular testing enables a rapid diagnosis, has higher sensitivity and specificity than AFB smear, and is able to distinguish *Mtb* from nontuberculous mycobacteria. One assay, the Xpert MTB/RIF (Gene Xpert, Sunnyvale, CA), detects *Mtb* DNA as well as mutations that confer resistance to rifampin. Gene Xpert is thus globally recommended as the initial diagnostic test for patients suspected of TB disease, including those with HIV co-infection. If the NAAT initially performed on a patient's sample detected the presence of *Mtb* DNA but did not also assess potential drug resistance, the sample testing positive should be sent immediately to a commercial or public health laboratory for molecular detection of drug resistance using Gene Xpert or similar assay.

In a patient with compatible clinical findings, a positive NAAT (or Gene Xpert) confirms TB diagnosis regardless of whether the smear is AFB positive or negative. If the AFB smear is positive but the NAAT is negative, then TB disease is unlikely. However, a negative AFB smear with negative NAAT does not rule out TB disease as false-negative results may occur, especially with paucibacillary disease often found in patients with HIV. Mycobacterial culture and growth-based DST should also be routinely performed regardless of the smear and NAAT results.

If rifampin resistance is detected, the patient's sample should be immediately sent to a laboratory that performs extended molecular detection of drug resistance (MDDR) (e.g., the Center for Disease Control and Prevention's (CDC's) TB Laboratory) to identify mutations associated with other first- and second-line TB drugs. If samples are sent expeditiously, results will be available to guide appropriate treatment within a very short time frame. Of note, molecular testing can also be performed on nonrespiratory samples in certain laboratories, which can be identified through your PHD or one of the regional TB Centers of Excellence (TB COE; https://www.cdc.gov/tb/education/tb_coe/default.htm) funded by the CDC.

Treatment of TB in Persons Living With HIV

Patients who are seriously ill should have TB therapy initiated as soon as possible (Table 17.1). If molecular DST indicates rifampin resistance within a few days of treatment initiation, adjustments can be safely made with little risk of acquired drug resistance. However, if molecular DST is not initially done and recognition of drug resistance is delayed, additional drug resistance can develop. For patients who are clinically stable at presentation, TB treatment can safely be deferred a day or so while waiting for molecular DST results to guide appropriate therapy. If rifampin resistance is detected, consult an expert in managing drug-resistant TB through the state or local PHD or one of the TB COEs.

Drug-susceptible TB is treated essentially the same in patients with and without HIV. The initial 2-month intensive phase consists of 4 drugs (rifampin, isoniazid, pyrazinamide, and ethambutol), followed by a 4-month continuation phase using only isoniazid and rifampin (Table 17.1). Daily therapy is preferred throughout treatment as highly intermittent therapy increases the risk of treatment failure or acquired rifampin resistance in patients with HIV. Most patients with HIV can be cured with a 6-month regimen, although TB treatment duration is extended for certain patients, especially those who are not receiving antiretroviral therapy (ART). Patients with central nervous system (CNS) involvement require adjunctive corticosteroids to avoid complications related to immune reconstitution.

TB treatment is given as directly observed therapy (DOT) by the PHD with close monitoring and patient-centered case management. Close collaboration between TB and HIV providers is also essential. Most patients can be released from isolation if they have been on appropriate TB therapy for 14 days, are clinically improving, and have 3 consecutive AFB-negative sputum smears.

Using ART During TB Treatment

Rifampin and rifabutin have activity against both actively replicating organisms and semidormant ("latent") mycobacteria and thus enable shortening TB treatment; without rifamycin, 18–24 months of TB therapy may be required. Rifampin is a potent inducer of metabolizing enzymes (e.g., CYP3A and CYP2B6) and drug transporters (e.g., P-glycoprotein) that decreases the plasma concentrations and effectiveness of many antiretroviral agents. Rifabutin is a weaker inducer of metabolizing enzymes but is also a CYP3A substrate, requiring a dose adjustment when given with strong CYP3A inducers or inhibitors. To avoid prolonged TB treatment,

TABLE 17.1 Treatment of Tuberculosis Disease in Patients With HIV Co-infection

TB Drug Regimens

	Intensive Phase	Duration: 8 Weeks	Continuation Phase	Duration: 18 Weeks
Regimen 1 (Preferred)	INH[a] RIF[b] (or RFB[c]) PZA[d] EMB[e]	Daily given by DOT • 5 days/week for 40 doses or • 7 days/week for 56 doses	INH[a] RIF[b] (or RFB[c])	Daily given by DOT • 5 days/week for 90 doses or • 7 days/week for 126 doses
Regimen 2 (Acceptable if daily DOT not feasible during continuation phase)	INH[a] RIF[b] (or RFB[c]) PZA[d] EMB[e]	Duration: 8 weeks Daily, given • 5 days/week for 40 doses or • 7 days/week for 56 doses	INH[f] RIF[g]	Intermittent, given 3 times weekly for 54 doses

TB Medication Dosage

DAILY

INH[a] 5 mg/kg (usual dose 300 mg)
RIF[b] 10 mg/kg (usual dose 600 mg)
RFB[c] 5 mg/kg (typically 300 mg)
PZA[d] Weight-based dosing
- *Weighing 40–55 kg:* 1000 mg (18.2–25.0 mg/kg)
- *Weighing 56–75 kg:* 1500 mg (20.0–26.8 mg/kg)
- *Weighing 76–90 kg:* 2000 mg (22.2–26.3 mg/kg)
- *Weighing > 90 kg:* 2000 mg[e]

EMB[e] Weight-based dosing
- *Weighing 40–55 kg:* 800 mg (14.5–20.0 mg/kg)
- *Weighing 56–75 kg:* 1200 mg (16.0–21.4 mg/kg)
- *Weighing 76–90 kg:* 1600 mg (17.8–21.1 mg/kg)
- *Weighing > 90 kg:* 1600 mg[e]

THRICE WEEKLY

INH[f] 15 mg/kg (typically 900 mg)
RIF[g] 10 mg/kg (typically 600mg)
RFB Not recommended for intermittent dosing
PZA[h] Weight-based dosing
- *Weighing 40–55 kg:* 1500 mg (27.3–37.5 mg/kg)
- *Weighing 56–75 kg:* 2500 mg (33.3–44.6 mg/kg)
- *Weighing 76–90 kg:* 3000 mg (33.3–39.5 mg/kg)
- *Weighing > 90 kg:* 4000 mg[e]

EMB[i] Weight-based dosing
- *Weighing 40–55 kg:* 1200 mg (21.8–30.0 mg/kg)
- *Weighing 56–75 kg:* 2000 mg (26.7–35.7) mg/kg)
- *Weighing 76–90 kg:* 2400 mg (26.7–31.6 mg/kg)
- *Weighing > 90 kg:* 1600 mg[e]

TABLE 17.1 **Continued**

TB Drug Regimens

Abbreviations: DOT, directly observed therapy; EMB, ethambutol; HIV, human immunodeficiency virus; INH, isoniazid; PZA, pyrazinamide; RFB, rifabutin; RIF, rifampin.

- Standard doses are listed and do not include adjustments for specific drug interactions.
- Give daily pyridoxine (25–50 mg B_6) to all patients with HIV taking INH since peripheral neuropathy is common in this population.
- Adjust the dose of PZA and EMB in patients with renal insufficiency or end-stage renal disease. INH and RIF do not require adjustment with renal disease.
- Therapeutic drug monitoring of serum drug concentrations may be useful for patients with HIV, especially those taking intermittent TB therapy and those with underlying renal disease, diabetes, and other risk of malabsorption.
- Other TB treatment regimens may be appropriate in certain circumstances; additional details and dosing recommendations for antiretroviral drugs with rifampin or rifamycin are shown in Table 17.2 or are available online https://www.cdc.gov/tb/publications/guidelines/pdf/Clin-Infect-Dis.-2016-Nahid-cid_ciw376.pdf or https://aidsinfo.nih.gov/guidelines/html/1/adult-and-adolescent-arv/0

Selected Guidelines for TB Treatment in Patients Living With HIV
Note: Recommendations are rated according to the criteria established in the Guidelines for the Prevention and Treatment of Opportunistic Infections in Adults and Adolescents with HIV (https://aidsinfo.nih.gov/guidelines/html/4/adult-and-adolescent-opportunistic-infection/325/mycobacterium-tuberculosis, accessed January 20, 2020).

- After collection of available specimens for culture and molecular diagnostic tests, empiric treatment for TB is warranted in patients with clinical and radiographic presentation suggestive of HIV-related TB (AIII).
- Treatment of suspected TB for individuals with HIV is the same as for individuals without HIV and should include an initial 4-drug combination of isoniazid, rifampin, ethambutol, and pyrazinamide (AI).
- DOT is recommended for all patients with suspected HIV-related TB (AII).
- Drug-susceptible TB should be treated with a 2-month intensive phase of the 4 drugs listed in the preceding item (isoniazid, rifampin, ethambutol, and pyrazinamide). Ethambutol can be discontinued when susceptibility to isoniazid and rifampin has been confirmed. Thereafter, isoniazid and a rifamycin are used in the continuation phase of therapy, generally recommended as an additional 4 months of treatment for uncomplicated TB (AI).

Continued

TABLE 17.1 **Continued**

TB Drug Regimens

- Although intermittent dosing (administration less often than daily) of anti-TB treatment facilitates DOT, regimens that included twice- or thrice-weekly dosing during the intensive or continuation phase have been associated with an increased risk of treatment failure or relapse with acquired drug resistance to the rifamycin class, particularly in persons living with HIV. Therefore, daily therapy given as DOT is recommended during both the intensive and the continuation treatment phases **(AII)**
- *Total Duration of Therapy:*

Pulmonary, drug-susceptible TB: 6 months **(BII)**

Pulmonary TB and positive culture at 2 months of TB treatment, severe cavitary disease, or disseminated extrapulmonary TB: 9 months **(BII)**

Extrapulmonary TB with CNS involvement: 9 to 12 months **(BII)**

Extrapulmonary TB in other sites: 6 months **(BII)**

- Adjunctive corticosteroid therapy is recommended in individuals with HIV who have TB involving the CNS **(AI)**. The regimen used in trials of adjunctive corticosteroids for CNS disease were dexamethasone (0.3–0.4 mg/kg/day for 2–4 weeks, then taper 0.1 mg/kg per week until a dose of 0.1 mg/kg, then 4 mg per day and taper by 1 mg/week; total duration of 12 weeks).
- Please note that while these doses above may be sufficient, there is no single established dose of steroids appropriate for all patients. Additionally, there is a drug-drug interaction between rifamycins and steroids (rifampin>>rifabutin) such that higher doses of steroids may be required to reduce signs and symptoms arising from the host immune reaction against *M. tuberculosis* antigens, especially when there is CNS disease. Steriod dose should be tailored to the individual patient's response to treatment, and the taper should be conducted slowly over months rather than weeks. If symptoms or signs recur during the taper, increase steroids again for a week or two then restart the taper slowly to maintain resolution of symptoms.
- Adjunctive corticosteroid therapy *is not recommended* in the treatment of TB pericarditis **(AI)**.
- ART should not be withheld until completion of TB treatment **(AI)**.
- ART is recommended for all persons with HIV and TB **(AI)**. For ART-naïve patients, ART should be started within 2 weeks after TB treatment initiation in those with CD4 count < 50 cells/mm^3 and, based on the preponderance of data, when TB meningitis is not suspected, within 8 weeks of starting anti-TB treatment in those with higher CD4 cell counts **(AI)**.

TABLE 17.1 **Continued**

TB Drug Regimens

- When TB occurs in patients already on ART, treatment for TB must be started immediately **(AIII)**, and ART should be modified to reduce the risk for drug interactions and maintain virologic suppression.
  - Paradoxical reaction (immune reconstitution inflammatory syndrome, IRIS) that is not severe may be treated symptomatically **(CIII)**.
  - For moderately severe paradoxical reaction, use of corticosteroid may be considered. Taper over 4 weeks (or longer) based on clinical symptoms **(BIII)**.
  - Preemptive prednisone therapy should be offered for high-risk patients with a CD4 count ≤ 100/mm³ who are starting ART in the context of recently initiated anti-TB therapy, are responding well to TB therapy, and who do not have rifampin resistance, Kaposi sarcoma, or active hepatitis B **(BI)**.

Examples of Prednisone Dosing Strategies for IRIS
- In patients on a rifampin-based regimen: prednisone 1.5 mg/kg/day for 2 weeks, then 0.75 mg/kg for 2 weeks
- In patients on a rifabutin plus boosted protease inhibitor–based regimen: prednisone 1.0 mg/kg/day for 2 weeks, then 0.5 mg/kg/day for 2 weeks
- A more gradual tapering schedule over a few months may be necessary in some patients.
  - Preemptive prednisone regimen: 40 mg/day for 2 weeks, then 20 mg/day for 2 weeks

TB-HIV treatment should include either an ART regimen that has no clinically significant drug interactions with rifampin or substitution of rifabutin for rifampin with appropriate ART and rifabutin dosing adjustments (Table 17.2).

Treatment decisions for TB-HIV must balance factors such as large pill burden, increased intolerance, overlapping toxicities, and risk of immune reconstitution inflammatory syndrome (IRIS) with risk of progressive immunosuppression, new opportunistic infections, and increased HIV-related mortality. If a patient is already taking ART when TB is diagnosed, initiate TB therapy and continue ART with appropriate adjustments to avoid drug interactions. For HIV treatment-naïve patients, TB treatment should be started as soon as possible, followed by ART within 2 to 8 weeks later, depending on the patient's level of immunosuppression. If the CD4 count

TABLE 17.2 **Drug-Drug Interactions Between Rifamycins and Antiretroviral Therapy**

Rifampin-Based TB Regimen With ART[a]

- *Nucleoside Reverse Transcriptase Inhibitors (NRTIs)*
  - Avoid rifampin with TAF-containing regimens if possible[b]
- *Non-Nucleoside Reverse Transcriptase Inhibitors (NNRTIs)*
  - Do not use EFV 400 mg with rifampin. Maintain EFV dose at 600 mg once daily and monitor for virologic response. Consider TDM.
  - Do not use rifampin with DOR, ETR, NVP, or RPV.
- *Protease Inhibitors (PIs)*
  - Do not use rifampin with any PI-containing regimen (boosted or unboosted).
- *Integrase Strand Transfer Inhibitors (INSTIs)*
  - Increase DTG to 50 mg twice daily; use alternative to rifampin, such as rifabutin, in patients with certain suspected or documented INSTI-associated resistance mutations.
  - Increase RAL to 800 mg twice daily; do not co-administer RAL 1200 mg once daily with rifampin. Monitor closely for virologic response or consider using rifabutin as an alternative to rifamycin.
  - Do not combine rifampin with BIC-containing regimens.
  - Do not use rifampin with EVG-containing regimens.
- *CCR5 Inhibitors*
  - Use MVC 600 mg twice daily if used *without* a strong CYP3A inhibitor:
  - Consider alternative ARV if used *with* a strong CYP3A inhibitor.

Rifabutin-Based TB Regimen With ART

- *NRTIs*
  - Avoid rifabutin with TAF-containing regimens if possible.[b]
- *NNRTIs*

NNRTI	Rifabutin
○ DOR	○ Increase DOR to 100 mg twice daily ○ Rifabutin 5 mg/kg once daily (usual dose 300 mg)
○ EFV	○ EFV 600 mg once daily ○ Rifabutin 450–600 mg once daily; or rifabutin 600 mg 3 times/week if EFV is not co-administered with a PI
○ ETR	○ ETR standard dose ○ Rifabutin 5 mg/kg once daily (usual dose 300 mg); do not use rifabutin if ETR given with RTV-boosted PI

TABLE 17.2 **Continued**

Rifampin-Based TB Regimen With ART[a]

- NVP
  - NVP standard dose
  - Rifabutin 5 mg/kg once daily (usual dose 300 mg)

- RPV
  - Increase RPV to 50 mg once daily
  - Rifabutin 5 mg/kg once daily (usual dose 300 mg)

- *PIs*

Ritonavir (/r)-boosted PIs[c] (do not use rifabutin with COBI-boosted regimens)

- Atazanavir (ATV)/r · Rifabutin 150 mg once daily; consider TDM

- Darunavir (DRV)/r

- Lopinavir/r

Unboosted PIs

- ATV
  - Rifabutin 150 mg once daily

- *INSTIs*
  - No dosage adjustments for DTG or rifabutin[d]
  - No dosage adjustments for RAL or rifabutin[d]
  - Do not combine rifabutin with BIC-containing regimens
  - Do not combine rifabutin with EVG-containing regimens
- *CCR5 Inhibitor*
  - MVC 150 mg twice daily (with strong CYP3A inhibitor);
  - MVC 300 mg twice daily (without strong CYP3A inhibitor or inducer);
  - Dose rifabutin based on other drugs in regimen (consider TDM).

Abbreviations: ART, antiretroviral therapy; BIC, bictegravir; COBI, cobicistat; DOR, doravirine; DTG, dolutegravir; EFV, efavirenz; ETR, etravirine; EVG, elvitegravir; EVG/c, elvitegravir/cobicistat; FTC, emtricitabine; HIV, human immunodeficiency virus; INSTI, integrase strand transfer inhibitor; MVC, maraviroc; NVP, nevirapine; PI, protease inhibitor; PK, pharmacokinetic; RAL, raltegravir; RIF, rifampin; RPV, rilpivirine; RTV, ritonavir; TAF, tenofovir alafenamide; TB, tuberculosis; TDM, therapeutic drug monitoring.

For the most current information on drug interactions, go to https://aidsinfo.nih.gov/contentfiles/lvguidelines/adult_oi.pdf (accessed January 20, 2020).

[a]All regimens use a standard rifampin dose of 600 mg. Isoniazid, pyrazinamide, and ethambutol do not require dose adjustment with any antiretroviral drug.

[b]A recent study suggested that TAF may be given together with rifampicin-containing TB treatment without dose adjustment. Caution is urged, however, as this combination has not been tested in patients to confirm PK and virologic efficacy among patients taking full-dose ART and TB regimens. Neither TDF nor TAF has been tested with rifabutin or rifapentine.

[c]All boosted PIs are standard dose.

[d]If a boosted PI is included in the regimen, see dosing recommendations listed above.

Source: Table reprinted from the "Treatment of Tuberculosis (TB) in Adults With HIV Infection" pocket card (https://sntc.medicine.ufl.edu/home/index#/products/94) with the permission of the Southeast National Tuberculosis Center and the Southeast AIDS Education and Training Center.

is less than 50/mm³, ART should be started within 2 weeks, and the patient should be closely monitored for adverse events, including IRIS. If the CD4 is 50/mm³ or greater, ART can be deferred for 8 weeks. If TB meningitis is present, ART should be held for the first 8–10 weeks of TB treatment regardless of the patient's CD4 count. Adjunctive corticosteroids are recommended for patients with HIV-related TB involving the CNS and may be beneficial in other select situations to avoid complications caused by enlarging lesions.

Treatment-Associated Adverse Events

Most patients tolerate TB treatment well regardless of HIV status. Nonetheless, some report gastrointestinal complaints; mild, transient rashes; joint pain; myalgia; headaches; or malaise, which can be symptomatically treated without stopping TB treatment. More severe dermatologic, hepatic, neurologic, hematologic, and other abnormalities can occur during treatment of either TB or HIV. Some drug-related adverse events do not affect the strength or duration of the regimen. For example, if ethambutol-related visual changes occur, treatment can be continued without substitution or extension as ethambutol has only weak activity against *Mtb*. In contrast, every effort should be made to maintain either rifampin or rifabutin in the TB regimen to avoid prolonged and inadequate therapy.

Hepatotoxicity is a potential side effect of several TB medications, ART, as well as TB and HIV diseases themselves. Patients should be evaluated at baseline and closely monitored during TB treatment to avoid this complication. TB treatment should be held if there is (1) increased bilirubin, (2) alanine aminotransferase (ALT) 3 times or greater the upper limit of normal (ULN) if symptoms are present, or (3) ALT 5 times or more the ULN even without symptoms. Other etiologies should be pursued, such as infection with hepatitis A, B, and C; gallbladder disease; underlying cirrhosis or fatty liver; and use of alcohol, acetaminophen, or other hepatotoxic substances. If no other cause is determined, drug-induced liver injury may be present.

If the patient cannot tolerate a short treatment interruption, a liver-gentle "bridging regimen" can be used, including drugs such as ethambutol, levofloxacin, cycloserine, or linezolid. Rifampin and ethambutol can be restarted when the ALT falls to less than 2 times the ULN or the bilirubin normalizes. After a week, either isoniazid or pyrazinamide can be rechallenged. If pyrazinamide is tolerated, isoniazid is not necessary as long as rifampin, ethambutol, and pyrazinamide are given for 6 months. If pyrazinamide cannot be added back but isoniazid is tolerated, TB therapy must be extended to 9 months. If one of the antiretroviral drugs is the cause of toxicity, appropriate substitutions should be made to maintain viral suppression.

Immune reconstitution inflammatory syndrome is another complication of TB-HIV treatment, resulting from an excessive local or systemic immune response against *Mtb* organisms in the setting of virologic response to ART. "Paradoxical" IRIS manifests as a worsening of clinical or radiographic findings after several weeks or months of improvement on treatment. Patients may experience new or recurrent symptoms, hectic fevers, enlarging adenopathy, worsening pleural effusion or infiltrates, and other abnormalities. With "unmasking" IRIS, new TB disease or sites of disease become evident after initiation of ART. Providers should be alert for serious complications of IRIS, such as enlarging cerebral tuberculomas, meningitis, pericardial effusions with cardiac tamponade, respiratory failure, airway obstruction, or splenic rupture. Both TB and ART treatment are continued in most cases, and most IRIS symptoms improve with symptomatic and anti-inflammatory therapies. Steroids may be needed to treat severe or life-threatening manifestations, and some high-risk patients may benefit from preemptive steroids (Table 17.1). IRIS is a diagnosis of exclusion, so patients should also be evaluated for new opportunistic infections, drug resistance, malabsorption, or nonadherence causing inadequate TB drug levels or drug toxicity.

Therapeutic drug monitoring and expert consultation can be used to ensure the safest, most effective treatment is used for both TB and HIV.

PREVENTION OF TB DISEASE

At the initial HIV clinical encounter, all patients should be evaluated for TB disease and tested for *Mtb* infection using either a TST or IGRA. Screening for new or ongoing TB exposure risk should be conducted annually and TST or IGRA repeated only if TB risk is present. TST or IGRA testing should be repeated if the initial test was performed when the CD4 count was less than 200 cells/mm^3 and has subsequently risen over 200 cells/

mm^3 after starting ART. Although either test is acceptable, IGRAs have higher specificity than TST (i.e., no cross-reactivity with prior BCG vaccination and most nontuberculous mycobacterial infections), do not require a second visit to read the result, and there is less subjectivity in determining a positive result. The sensitivity of both tests decreases with worsening immunosuppression.

THE PATIENT IN THIS CASE LIVES WITH HER HUSBAND, WHO IS ALSO LIVING WITH HIV

What Do You Do Now?

As a close contact to an infectious person, the husband should be carefully evaluated to ensure he does not already have TB disease. If he has no symptoms, a chest x-ray is normal, and he has a positive TST (>5-mm induration) or IGRA, he can be diagnosed as having LTBI. For patients with LTBI and HIV co-infection, early initiation of ART substantially reduces the risk of TB disease at any CD4 cell count, although risk remains 3–12 times above that of the general population. LTBI treatment is also effective for preventing TB disease, and the effect is highest when combined with ART.

This man should be treated with an appropriate LTBI regimen, which can reduce his risk of developing active disease by approximately 80% if he completes treatment (Box 17.1). Even if his TST and IGRA were negative, preventive treatment is warranted since he has known TB exposure and his TST or IGRA could be falsely negative.

Isoniazid is most often used for patients with HIV and LTBI because it has no known drug interactions with ART and is relatively safe. Because isoniazid is a 9-month regimen, poor treatment completion rates undermine its effectiveness. Two shorter rifamycin-based LTBI regimens are also recommended: (1) once-weekly isoniazid and rifapentine ("3HP") given 12 weeks by DOT (preferred) or self-administered and (2) daily rifampin monotherapy self-administered for 4 months. Both of these rifamycin-based regimens have been shown noninferior to 9 months of isoniazid, and both have lower risk of hepatotoxicity and higher treatment completion

Indications for LTBI Treatment

- (+) TST or IGRA, no evidence of TB disease, and no prior history of treatment for TB disease or LTBI
- Close contact with a person with infectious TB, regardless of TST or IGRA result

LTBI Treatment Regimens:

Use with any ART regimen:

- Isoniazid monotherapy[a]: INH 300 mg daily + B_6 25–50 mg daily for 9 months by SAT

Use only if not receiving ART or receiving an EFV- or RAL-based ART regimen without TAF.

- Isoniazid/rifapentine[b] "3HP": INH 15 mg/kg weekly (900 mg maximum) + RPT weight based (see next), 900 mg maximum weekly + B_6 50 mg weekly for 12 weeks
  - if weight 32.1–49.9 kg, use RPT 750 mg
  - if weight ≥ 50.0 kg, use RPT 900 mg
- Rifampin monotherapy: RIF 600 mg daily for 4 months given by SAT
  - Substitute rifabutin daily for 4 months by SAT if RIF cannot be used due to drug-drug interactions. RFB dose adjusted based on concomitant ART (see Table 17.2)

Abbreviations: ART, antiretroviral therapy; B_6, pyridoxine; DOT, directly observed therapy; EFV, efavirenz; IGRA, interferon gamma release assay; INH, isoniazid; LTBI, latent tuberculosis infection; RAL, raltegravir; RFB, rifabutin; RIF, rifampin; RPT, rifapentine; SAT, self-administered therapy; TAF, tenofovir alafenamide; TB, tuberculosis; TST, tuberculin skin test.

Note: Rifamycins (RIF, RBT, and RPT) cannot be used with TAF.

All LTBI regimens are given orally

[a]Isoniazid is not recommended for pregnant women with LTBI until after delivery unless they are close contacts of a known patient with active TB disease.

[b]Preferably give 3HP by DOT. 3HP can be given by SAT in select patients who demonstrated good adherence to the first 2–3 doses (contact an TB-HIV expert).

For additional information on potential drug-drug interactions during TB-HIV treatment, see https://www.hiv-druginteractions.org ; https://aidsinfo.nih.gov/guidelines/html/4/adult-and-adolescent-opportunistic-infection/0; or https://aidsinfo.nih.gov/guidelines/html/1/adult-and-adolescent-arv/0

Table reprinted from the "Treatment of Tuberculosis (TB) in Adults with HIV Infection" pocket card (https://sntc.medicine.ufl.edu/home/index#/products/94) with the permission of the Southeast National Tuberculosis Center and the Southeast AIDS Education and Training Center.

rates. Both are limited by potential drug interactions with ART and are only recommended for patients who either are not taking ART or are taking efavirenz- or raltegravir-based regimens and that do not include tenofovir alafenamide. A 1-month daily regimen of rifapentine plus isoniazid (1HP) was recently found noninferior to 9 months of isoniazid for preventing HIV-related TB, but this regimen has not yet been recommended in national or global guidelines.

KEY POINTS TO REMEMBER

- Pulmonary and extrapulmonary TB disease can occur at any CD4 cell count and requires a high index of suspicion.
- Patients with pulmonary involvement may be infectious to others and should be isolated at home or in a health facility.
- Diagnosis of pulmonary TB disease should include testing 3 sputum specimens for AFB smear, mycobacterial culture, and DST; at least one should be tested using molecular methods that detect *M. tuberculosis* and rifampin resistance.
- TB disease is treated using a 2-month intensive phase with rifampin, isoniazid, pyrazinamide, and ethambutol, followed by a 4-month continuation phase using only rifampin and isoniazid; some patients with HIV may require longer therapy.
- Patients with HIV and LTBI should be evaluated for active pulmonary and extrapulmonary TB, then treated with both LTBI preventive therapy and ART.
- Screening tests (TST and IGRA) cannot distinguish TB disease from LTBI and can be falsely negative in immunosuppressed patients.

ACKNOWLEDGMENT

We would like to thank Dr. David Ashkin (University of Miami and Southeast National Tuberculosis Center at the University of Florida) for reviewing this chapter.

Further Reading

Borisov AS, Bamrah Morris S, Gibril JN, et al. Update of recommendations for use of once-weekly isoniazid-rifapentine regimen to treat latent *Mycobacterium tuberculosis* infection. *MMWR Morb Mortal Wkly Rep*. 2018;67(25):723–726.

Griesel R, Stewart A, Van der Plas H, et al. Optimizing tuberculosis diagnosis in human immunodeficiency virus-infected inpatients meeting the criteria of seriously ill in the World Health Organization algorithm. *Clin Infec Dis*. 2018;66(9):1419–1426.

Lewinsohn DM, Leonard MK, LoBue PA, et al. Official American Thoracic Society/ Infectious Diseases Society of America/Centers for Disease Control and Prevention clinical practice guidelines: diagnosis of tuberculosis in adults and children. *Clin Infect Dis*. 2017;64(2):111–115.

Meintjes G, Stek C, Blumenthal L, et al. (2018). Prednisone for the prevention of paradoxical tuberculosis-associated IRIS. *N Engl J Med*. 2018;379:1915–1925.

Nahid P, Dorman SE, Alipanah N, et al. Official American Thoracic Society/Centers for Disease Control and Prevention/Infectious Diseases Society of America clinical practice guidelines: treatment of drug-susceptible tuberculosis. *Clin Infect Dis*. 2016;63(7):e147–e195.

Panel on Opportunistic Infections in Adults and Adolescents With HIV. Guidelines for the prevention and treatment of opportunistic infections in adults and adolescents with HIV: recommendations from the Centers for Disease Control and Prevention, the National Institutes of Health, and the HIV Medicine Association of the Infectious Diseases Society of America. http://aidsinfo.nih.gov/ contentfiles/lvguidelines/adult_oi.pdf. Accessed January, 20, 2020.

Sterling TR, Njie G, Zenner D, et al. Guidelines for the treatment of latent tuberculosis infection: recommendations from the National Tuberculosis Controllers Association and CDC. *MMWR Recomm Rep*. 2020;69(1):1–11.

Swindells S, Ramchandani R, Gupta A, et al. (2019). One month of rifapentine plus isoniazid to prevent HIV-related tuberculosis. *N Engl J Med*. 2019;380(11):1001–1011.

Tornheim JA, Dooley KE. Tuberculosis associated with HIV infection. *Microbiol Spectr*. 2017;5(1). doi:10.1128/microbiolspec.TNMI7-0028-2016

18 "I've got a bad headache"

Khalil Nasser and Moti Ramgopal

A 24-year-old woman with a history of HIV presents to
the emergency room with worsening headache over
the past 4 days without any nausea or vomiting. The
headaches have been intermittent for several months
but have now progressively worsened. Her speech
is normal; she denies head trauma, syncope, loss of
consciousness, chest pains, shortness of breath, or
blurred vision. Medications include darunavir/cobicistat,
emtricitabine/tenofovir disoproxil fumarate, and
trimethoprim-sulfamethoxazole (TMP/SMX), however,
though she has been off antiretroviral therapy (ART)
for several years due cost issues. She attends college
full time and works part-time at a fast food restaurant,
making it difficult for her to see her primary provider.

On physical examination, she is febrile at 100.9°F. There is
no oral thrush, pupils are reactive to light bilaterally, lungs
are clear to auscultation bilaterally, cranial nerves II–XII
are preserved, there are no meningeal signs, and no focal
neurological deficits are observed. Her most recent CD4+ was
27. A urine pregnancy test was negative.

What Do You Do Now?

HEADACHE IN A PATIENT LIVING WITH HIV WITH A LOW CD4+

When evaluating and managing an HIV patient presenting with headache, it is important to differentiate patients into categories based on CD4+ cell count with and without intracranial lesions. Patients presenting with headache and central nervous system (CNS) lesions with low CD4+ count, most common diagnostic infections are toxoplasmosis, lymphoma, and progressive multifocal leukoencephalopathy (PML). For headaches in HIV without CNS lesions, the most common diagnostic infections are cryptococcosis, herpes simplex virus (HSV), and cytomegalovirus (CMV). Neurosyphilis, which can occur at any CD4+ count and at any stage of syphilis among persons living with HIV (PLWH), should be suspected if there is evidence of neurologic symptoms, including ophthalmologic or auditory signs.

In this case, a 24-year-old woman with HIV/AIDS, off ART for several years with last CD4+ count at 27 cells/µL, presents with progressively worsening headache for several months. She was febrile on admission, later testing negative for both serum cryptococcal antigen and serum Venereal Disease Research Laboratory (VDRL) text. Contrast-enhanced head computed tomography (CT) showed no mass effect, but multiple ring-enhancing lesions were found in the cerebellum bilaterally, basal ganglia, and corticomedullary junction as well as mastoiditis. At this point, the differential diagnosis includes toxoplasmosis, lymphoma, bacterial/fungal abscess, primary brain tumor, brain metastasis from systemic cancer, tuberculoma, and lesions of fungal origin.

A serum toxoplasma immunoglobulin (Ig) G test was positive, with a negative toxoplasma IgM, so the patient was later started on empiric treatment for toxoplasmosis with pyrimethamine 100 mg for 1 day as a loading dose, then 25 to 50 mg per day, plus sulfadiazine 2 to 4 g daily for 2 days, followed by a 500-mg to 1-gdose 4 times per day, plus folinic acid 5–25 mg with each dose of pyrimethamine for a planned 4 to 6 weeks of therapy, followed by revaluation of the patient's condition. She was evaluated for reinitiation of ART 2 weeks after starting empiric treatment for toxoplasmosis and started on combination bictegravir 50 mg, emtricitabine 200 mg, and tenofovir alafenamide 25 mg once daily.

Pyrimethamine, considered the most effective drug against toxoplasmosis, is a folic acid antagonist and can cause dose-related suppression of the bone marrow, which is mitigated by concurrent administration of folinic acid. In patients with sulfa allergy or intolerance, clindamycin and atovaquone are alternatives to sulfadiazine; however, use of clindamycin is associated with a slightly increased incidence of recrudescence. These combinations, however, do not prevent *Pneumocystis jirovecii* pneumonia (PJP; formerly *Pneumocystis carinii* pneumonia, PCP); therefore, additional PJP prophylaxis must be administered when it is used. Due to cost-prohibitive pricing of pyrimethamine in the United States, pyrimethamine may not be readily available. If pyrimethamine is unavailable, clinicians may substitute with TMP/SMX or atovaquone dosed according to age and weight.

Patients who have completed initial therapy for toxoplasmosis should be given chronic maintenance therapy to suppress infection until immune reconstitution occurs as a sequence of ART, in which case treatment discontinuation is indicated. The combination of pyrimethamine plus sulfadiazine plus leucovorin is highly effective as suppressive therapy for patients with toxoplasmosis and provides protection against PJP. Pyrimethamine plus clindamycin is commonly used as suppressive therapy for patients with toxoplasmosis who cannot tolerate sulfa drugs. Adults and adolescent patients receiving chronic maintenance therapy for toxoplasmosis are at low risk for recurrence if they have successfully completed initial therapy, remain asymptomatic, and have an increase in their CD4+ count to more than 200 cells/μL after ART that is sustained for more than 6 months. Discontinuing chronic maintenance therapy in such patients is a reasonable consideration, although occasional recurrences have been reported. As part of the evaluation to determine whether discontinuation of therapy is appropriate, some specialists recommend obtaining magnetic resonance imaging (MRI) of the brain to assess for resolution of brain lesions.

Following 6 weeks of empiric treatment for toxoplasmosis and 4 weeks of ART, CD4+ cells rose to 80 cells/μL. Follow-up examinations showed signs of lesion regression on CT scans and resolution of the patient's headache. She also had a rise in CD4+ count to 390 cells/μL 1 year following reinitiation of ART with HIV-1 viral load less than 20 copies/mL, at which point prophylaxis with TMP/SMX was discontinued. Like other opportunistic infections (OIs), toxoplasmosis is on the decline in the era of effective ART; however, nonadherence to ART and CD4-guided prophylaxis presents a significant challenge in the prevention of OIs in PLWH.

The incidence of nearly all AIDS-defining OIs decreased significantly in the post-ART era, with the most common OIs being PJP, esophageal candidiasis, and disseminated *Mycobacterium avium* complex (MAC) disease. PJP, the most common serious OI as an interstitial pneumonia, continues to occur primarily in persons not previously receiving medical care. The most profound effect on survival of PLWH is conferred by virologic suppression achieved on ART, but specific OI prevention measures are as well associated with a survival benefit, even when they coincide with the administration of ART. This decline in the incidence of OIs has left physicians less cognizant of the nuances of OI treatment in the present era.

What we have learned in the last 10–15 years is that early initiation of ART is associated with a decrease in HIV progression to death. For most PLWH with an acute OI, ART should be considered within the first 2 weeks of initiating treatment for the acute OI. However, in cryptococcus and mycobacterial diseases, it has been shown that there is increased mortality and morbidity with early initiation of ART. ART use in the treatment of OIs is complicated by drug interactions, drug toxicity profiles, and immune reconstitution inflammatory syndrome (IRIS).

Primary and secondary prophylaxis against OIs is essential in prevention of initial or recurrent episodes of OIs in PLWH. Prophylaxis against many OIs can usually be discontinued for patients who respond to ART and maintain CD4+ cells above the recommended threshold for more than 3 months. However, if the CD4+ cells decrease below that threshold, prophylaxis should be resumed. Continued monitoring of incidence trends and detection of new syndromes associated with ART are important priorities in the ART era. Here, we present cases of OIs we see most frequently today.

Cerebral toxoplasmosis is the most common cause of space-occupying intracranial focal mass lesions in PLWH and typically results from reactivation of latent infection of *Toxoplasma gondii*, an obligate intracellular parasite. Most *Toxoplasma* disease in PLWH occurs in patients who have a CD4+ count less than 100 cells/μL, at which point prophylaxis with TMP/SMX should be initiated. TMP/SMX also doubles as PJP prophylaxis when started at CD4+ less than 200 cells/μL, as PJP still represents the most common OI in PLHW. Imaging studies can also provide supportive information. MRI with or without contrast has greater sensitivity than contrast-enhanced CT, especially for detecting multiple lesions, subcortical lesions, and posterior fossa involvement. However, neither imaging modality alone is sufficient to make a diagnosis because there is no pathognomonic radiographically distinguishing feature of toxoplasmosis compared to primary CNS lymphoma (PCNSL).

Toxoplasmosis often presents with subacute changes in level of consciousness, fever, headaches, seizures, and/or focal neurologic deficits. Investigative studies such as cerebrospinal fluid (CSF) analysis toxoplasma serology or imaging studies do not always provide a definitive diagnosis. In this patient population, obtaining a lumbar puncture is often contraindicated due to the presence of lesions with mass effect and increased risk of herniation. In cases in which a CSF sample is obtained, analysis frequently shows nonspecific mild mononuclear pleocytosis with elevated protein. Polymerase chain reaction (PCR) can increase utility of CSF analysis. PCR can detect *T. gondii* with high specificity (100%) but variable sensitivity (30%–50%). Consequently, whereas a positive PCR result is highly suggestive of the diagnosis, a negative result does not exclude toxoplasmosis. Toxoplasmosis typically presents as multiple, homogeneous, ring-enhancing lesions with cerebral edema and mass effect. It has a predilection for the basal ganglia and corticomedullary junction, with involvement of both white and gray matter.

Although a solitary mass lesion with edema is often observed with PCNSL, it can also be seen in toxoplasmosis. Thallium single-photon emission computed tomography (SPECT) and positron emission tomography (PET) can be useful in distinguishing toxoplasmosis from lymphoma. Lymphoma has increased thallium uptake on SPECT and hypermetabolism of glucose and methionine on PET. *Toxoplasma* is hypometabolic on PET and does not show uptake on thallium. Biopsy is often pursued in patients who do not improve with empirical toxoplasmosis management, usually within 2 weeks, have large mass effect with impending herniation, or require a rapid definitive diagnosis.

In the United States, prior to the availability of effective ART, the incidence of *Toxoplasma* encephalitis among PLHW with CD4+ less than 100 cells/µL was 40 per 1000 person-years; this rate has decreased significantly with widespread use of ART and TMP/SMX for prophylaxis. In comparison, cryptococcosis commonly presents as a subacute meningitis or meningoencephalitis with fever, malaise, and headache. Classic meningeal symptoms and signs, such as neck stiffness and photophobia, occur in only one-quarter to one-third of patients. Some patients experience encephalopathic symptoms, such as lethargy, altered mentation, personality changes, and memory loss, which are usually a result of increased intracranial pressure (ICP). Meningeal cryptococcosis can lead to sudden catastrophic vision loss. Cryptococcosis usually is disseminated when diagnosed in PLWH.

Analysis of CSF generally demonstrates mildly elevated levels of serum protein, low-to-normal glucose concentrations, and pleocytosis consisting mostly of lymphocytes. Some PLWH will have very few CSF inflammatory cells, but a Gram stain preparation, or an India ink preparation if available, may demonstrate numerous yeast forms. The opening pressure in the CSF may be elevated, with pressures greater than 25 cm H_2O occurring in 60% to 80% of patients. An opening pressure must be documented because its elevation is associated with higher CSF fungal burden and also higher neurological morbidity and mortality.

Cryptococcal disease can be diagnosed through culture, CSF microscopy, or cryptococcal antigen (CrAg) detection. PCR-based diagnosis of cryptococcal meningitis has not been broadly adopted given the high sensitivity, wide availability, and low cost of CrAg testing, although it may be clinically useful as adjuvant testing using a multiplex meningitis/encephalitis PCR panel (FilmArray System, BioFire Diagnostics) to distinguish between relapsed disease and paradoxical IRIS.

In patients with HIV-related cryptococcal meningitis, 55% of blood cultures and 95% of CSF cultures are positive, and visible colonies can be detected within 7 days. India ink staining of CSF demonstrates encapsulated yeast in 60% to 80% of cases. Cryptococcal meningitis is a disease with a high organism burden and low inflammatory response, which thus leads to increased ICP due to failure of CSF absorption at the arachnoid villi. A positive serum CrAg should prompt a lumbar puncture to rule out meningeal disease.

Testing for the antigen in the serum is a useful initial screening tool in diagnosing suspected cryptococcosis in PLWH, and it may be particularly useful when a lumbar puncture is delayed or refused. Predictors of poor clinical outcome of cryptococcal meningitis in PLWH include low weight, CSF cryptococcal antigen titer greater than 1:1024, CSF white blood cells less than 20, abnormal mental status on presentation, and diastolic hypertension (reflective of increased ICP). Routine testing for serum CrAg in newly diagnosed PLWH with no overt clinical signs of meningitis is recommended by some experts for patients whose CD4+ counts are less than 100 cells/μL and particularly in those with CD4+ count less than 50 cells/μL, with overall CrAg prevalence by serum enzyme immunoassay of 3.6% (95% CI 2.0%–6.0%) with CD4+ less than 200 cells/μL, and 5.7% (95% CI 2.8%–10.2%) with CD4+ less than 100 cells/μL among PLWH in the Multicenter AIDS Cohort Study and the Women's Interagency HIV Study cohorts in the United States. Although, the Centers for Disease Control and Prevention does not currently require screening of individuals from certain countries, it is worth mentioning that the majority of worldwide cases occur in sub-Saharan Africa, Asia, and the Pacific.

Treating cryptococcosis consists of three phases: induction, consolidation, and maintenance therapy. The preferred therapy for cryptococcal meningitis is a combination of intravenous liposomal amphotericin B at 3–4 mg/kg daily in combination with oral flucytosine 100 mg/kg daily divided in 4 doses for 2 weeks followed by oral fluconazole 400 mg daily to complete 10 weeks of therapy during the consolidative phase. Lipid formulations of amphotericin B have been shown to be effective for disseminated cryptococcosis, particularly in patients who experience clinically significant renal dysfunction during therapy or who are likely to develop it. Elevations in ICP can be treated with repeat daily lumbar punctures for 4 to 7 days, with the goal of lowering ICP to less than 20 cm H_2O. If elevated ICP persists beyond 20–25 with symptoms, then a temporary percutaneous lumbar drain or ventriculostomy shunt can be used. The flucytosine dose must be adjusted in patients with renal impairment.

If flucytosine is not available or the patient experiences drug toxicity, the patient can be treated with a combination of amphotericin B with fluconazole either 400 mg or 800 mg once daily for 14 days. A repeat lumbar puncture should be done at the end of the 2-week period to document a negative CSF fungal culture. Intravenous amphotericin B should be continued if the patient has persistently positive CSF cultures, is clinically deteriorating or comatose, or has persistent elevated and symptomatic ICPs. Following serum cryptococcal antigen during treatment is also recommended.

In PLWH, sensitivity in serum is similar to sensitivity in CSF. During therapy for acute infection, an unchanged or increased titer of antigen in CSF has been correlated with clinical and microbiological failure to respond to treatment. Attempts to treat increased ICP with medication therapy, such as mannitol, acetazolamide, or corticosteroids, is not effective and is not recommended. A therapeutic lumbar puncture to decrease ICP was associated with a reduced risk of death in a study performed in Africa. The same study also documented that ART should be deferred until 5 weeks after initial presentation to avoid an increase in mortality by reducing the risk of IRIS in patients with cryptococcal meningitis. Several additional studies supported the approach of deferring ART for at least several weeks. Nonetheless, the optimal timing of ART is unclear, and clinicians who decide to initiate ART prior to week 10 in the course of treating cryptococcal meningitis should be prepared to aggressively address complications caused by IRIS, such as elevated ICP.

Immune reconstitution inflammatory syndrome occurs after the initiation of combination ART and either "unmasks" a previous subclinical infection or worsens a known infection despite appropriate therapy (paradoxical reaction). In the CNS, IRIS can develop with many opportunistic processes, most commonly cryptococcal meningitis, TB meningitis, and PML. Cryptococcal IRIS can develop between 1 and 10 months after initiating ART and can present as culture-negative meningitis, cryptococcomas, pneumonitis, and/or lymphadenopathy. Adjunctive steroids should be considered for refractory increased ICP.

Treatment of IRIS usually consists of continued treatment of the OI and HIV ART with use of nonsteroidal anti-inflammatory drugs (NSAIDs) and/or corticosteroids for symptomatic treatment of IRIS. NSAIDS are preferred, but systemic symptoms that are severe or cases with large inflammatory masses usually require steroids: prednisone 1–2 mg/kg per day for 1–2 weeks followed by tapering based on symptoms. Most patients show improvement within 3 days. In some cases, it is necessary to give prolonged courses, surgically resect masses, drain abscesses, or even stop treatment of HIV and/or OIs due to life-threatening IRIS.

Additionally, CD8+ T-cell encephalitis syndrome, a severe form of HIV-associated neurocognitive disorder (HAND), has been described in patients receiving ART with low or undetectable serum HIV viral loads. HAND is associated with significant cognitive, behavioral, and motor abnormalities that can impact ART compliance, retention in care in older individuals, virological success, and quality of life. Patients can present with HAND, headache, focal neurological deficits, new-onset seizures, status epilepticus, and altered mental status, with MRI of the brain showing bilateral white matter lesions. CSF usually shows a lymphocytic pleocytosis with CD8+ T cells greater than 65%. Patients improve dramatically with corticosteroids and with improved CNS penetration of their ART regimen. The optimal dose and duration of corticosteroids are currently unknown. Furthermore, HAND is associated with virological failure, and, when combined with frailty, it is associated with greater risk for falls, disability, and death.

Patients who have completed the first 10 weeks of induction and consolidation therapy for acute cryptococcosis should be given chronic maintenance or suppressive therapy with 200 mg of fluconazole daily. Discontinuation of antifungal maintenance treatment is recommended when patients are either (1) stable and adherent to ART and antifungal maintenance therapy for at least 1 year and show evidence of immune reconstitution with CD4+ cell count of greater than or equal to 200 cells/μL or (2) adherent to ART and antifungal maintenance treatment for at least 1 year and a CD4+ cell count of greater than or equal to 100 cells/μL and a suppressed viral load. Maintenance treatment for cryptococcal disease should be restarted if CD4+ count drops to 100 cells/μL or if a World Health Organization (WHO) Stage 4 clinical event occurs. The risk of relapsed cryptococcal meningitis is influenced by (1) the choice of induction therapy, with a higher mortality risk with fluconazole monotherapy, which can select for resistance; (2) nonadherence to or lack of secondary prophylaxis; and (3) failure of linkage to care or retention in care of HIV ART programs.

When a patient develops recurrent symptoms of meningitis, it is important to consider both IRIS and relapse in the differential diagnosis. It is clinically impossible to distinguish between IRIS and relapse based on symptoms alone. The critical distinguishing feature is a sterile CSF, which is more associated with paradoxical cryptococcal IRIS, rather than relapse.

It is important to differentiate between IRIS and cryptococcal relapse because the therapeutic approach differs depending on the etiology behind recurrent symptoms. Since there is no laboratory test available for detection of paradoxical cryptococcal meningitis IRIS, it remains primarily a clinical diagnosis of exclusion, with the principal consideration being exclusion of culture-positive relapse. A positive CSF culture for *Cryptococcus neoformans* is diagnostic for microbiologic relapse or treatment failure. Furthermore, CrAg titers are not precise indicators for early relapse or for making therapeutic decisions, although titers may be clinically helpful for determining late relapse. While not definitive, an unchanged or rising CrAg titer several months after initial cryptococcal meningitis diagnosis should raise one's suspicion for microbiologic relapse while one awaits the culture. CD4 is not a useful diagnostic marker for either cryptococcal meningitis IRIS or relapse. Data suggest that relapse rates can be anywhere between 6% and 23%.

The frequency of cryptococcosis in the pre-ART era was 5%–8% in PLWH. This OI has now become relatively rare in the United States and seen almost exclusively in those with a CD4+ count of less than 100 cells/μL. Current estimates indicate that every year, nearly 1 million cases of cryptococcal meningitis are diagnosed worldwide, and the disease accounts for more than 600,000 deaths. Despite this, the most common causes of meningitis in patients with advanced immunosuppression are *C. neoformans*, tuberculosis, and toxoplasmosis. As opposed to PLWH with profound immunosuppression, approximately one-third of patients with HIV who present with meningitis do so during the early stages of the HIV disease (i.e., CD4+ count greater than 200 cells/μL). The most common causes of meningitis in these patients are herpes simplex type 2, varicella zoster virus (VZV), and arboviruses (West Nile, St. Louis encephalitis).

PML, HSV, AND CMV ENCEPHALITIS

Progressive multifocal leukoencephalopathy is characterized by multifocal areas of demyelination caused by the John Cunningham (JC) virus. PML lesions are usually bilateral, asymmetric, and localized preferentially to the periventricular areas and the subcortical white matter. The lesions are generally not contrast enhancing and are not surrounded by edema; as a result, a substantial mass effect on surrounding structures is absent. Although usually seen in untreated PLWH with severe immunosuppression, PML may occur in the setting of IRIS, with a lower nadir CD4 considered a risk factor. In this context, PML/IRIS can present with contrast enhancement on MRI, as well as focal edema and mass effect. Patients with PML characteristically present with rapidly progressive focal neurologic deficits, including hemiparesis, visual field deficits, ataxia, aphasia, and cognitive impairment.

The clinical presentation of herpes encephalitis is often characterized by the rapid onset of fever, headache, seizures, focal neurologic signs, and impaired consciousness. Diagnosis can be determined with lumbar puncture for CSF analysis and PCR testing for HSV in any patient with encephalitis. MRI is recommended to assess signs of temporal lobe involvement, which would support the diagnosis. Absence of this finding does not alter decisions regarding empiric therapy. Brain MRI would also eliminate other alternative causes of mental status changes, such as brain abscess. Brain biopsy is recommended if the patient clinically deteriorates on appropriate therapy and PCR testing is negative for HSV. Treatment for suspected HSV encephalitis is recommended, with empiric therapy including acyclovir (10 mg/kg/ IV every 8 hours) for 14–21 days.

Cytomegalovirus encephalitis, caused by CMV with CD4+ less than 50 cells/µL, occurs in less than 0.5% of patients with AIDS. Two forms of CMV encephalitis are seen in patients with AIDS. One resembles HIV encephalitis and presents as progressive dementia; the other is a ventriculoencephalitis characterized by cranial nerve deficits, nystagmus, disorientation, lethargy, and ventriculomegaly. The former is characterized by multifocal, diffusely scattered micronodules widely distributed in the cortex, basal ganglia, brainstem, and cerebellum, while ventriculoencephalitis is characterized by progressive ventricular enlargement, periventricular enhancement, and increased periventricular signal on T2-weighted images. Rarely, CMV causes focal ring-enhancing lesions with edema and mass effect. Clinical features include rapidly progressive delirium, cranial nerve deficits, nystagmus, ataxia, and headache with fever

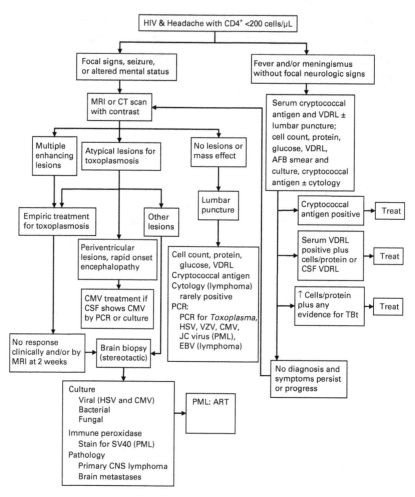

FIGURE 18.1 Diagnostic algorithm for headache in PLWH.

with or without CMV retinitis. Diagnosis can be supported with an MRI showing periventricular confluent lesions with enhancement. CMV PCR in CSF is greater than 80% sensitive and 90% specific, and cultures of CSF for CMV are usually negative. Treatment for CMV encephalitis includes a combination of ganciclovir 5 mg/kg IV every 12 hours, foscarnet 90 mg/kg IV every 12 hours, plus ART. Please review Figure 18.1 when examining OIs presenting as headache in PLWH.

· Lumbar puncture with PCR of CSF can rapidly detect HSV, toxoplasmosis, CMV, and JC virus.

· Cryptococcal meningitis induction treatment for 2 weeks should be completed before considering ART initiation, especially if ICP has normalized. In the setting of increased ICP after 2 weeks of low CSF white blood cells, delay of ART should be considered until completion of consolidation at 10 weeks.

· The most common focal mass lesion in PLWH is toxoplasmosis; prophylactic agents such as TMP-SMX can decrease the incidence of toxoplasmosis.

Further Reading

Bartlett J, Redfield R, Pham P. *Bartlett's Medical Management of HIV Infection*. 17th ed. New York, NY: Oxford University Press; 2019.

Bennett J, Dolin R, Blaser M, Mandell D. *Bennett's Principles and Practice of Infectious Diseases*. 3rd ed. Philadelphia, PA: Elsevier; 2015.

Kasper D, Fauci A. *Harrison's Infectious Diseases*. 3rd ed. New York, NY: McGraw Hill Education Medical; 2017.

Wright W. *Essentials of Clinical Infectious Diseases*. 2nd ed. New York, NY: Demos Medical; 2018.

19 "I feel pretty good, but my body is slowing down … "

Patricia Heaslip and Oluwatoyin M. Adeyemi

AJ, a 55-year-old black woman with HIV for 17 years, complains of fatigue. She notes her gait is slower, and she feels weak during normal activities. She states she forgets her appointments and sometimes other tasks. Medical history includes hepatitis C virus (HCV), diabetes mellitus, hypertension, peripheral neuropathy, hyperlipidemia, and smoking. She has been virally suppressed for the past 12 years following a CD4 nadir of 85 on antiretroviral therapy (ART) initiation. Currently, her CD4 value is 430. A lung nodule was incidentally noted 8 months ago on a chest x-ray, and she has missed several appointments for a mammogram and chest computed tomography (CT). She takes metformin, enalapril, nifedipine, atorvastatin, pantoprazole, gabapentin, trazodone, and supplements for energy. Her blood pressure is 102/66, and her body mass index is 30. Although obese, she has decreased muscle mass and has lost 10 kg since her last visit. She admits she has not been taking all of her medications due to difficulty reading the labels and forgetfulness. Her sister, who helps her, was recently diagnosed with cancer and is no longer able to provide supportive care.

What Do You Do Now?

THE AGING HIV PATIENT

The aging HIV patient presents unique and complex challenges that require multidisciplinary care. It is important to note that the duration of HIV infection is associated with a higher rate of frailty and comorbidities independent of age. The overlapping impact of lifestyle, HIV viremia, HIV medications, inflammation, immune activation, and illnesses of aging make the elderly population one that demands special attention. Almost half of all person living with HIV (PLWH) in the United States are aged 50 and older, and this number is expected to continue to rise. Knowing that PLWH have a life expectancy roughly within 5 to 10 years of their matched HIV uninfected peers, providers can expect to face multiple chronic comorbid conditions when caring for an aging patient with HIV.

Prior to combination antiretroviral therapy (cART), many PLWH have debilitating opportunistic infections and cancers, leaving preventive health screenings and chronic conditions much less of a concern. However, since HIV has become a more manageable chronic condition, the main determinants of overall health and quality of life are more likely to be related to the long-term consequences of chronic comorbid illnesses and less from HIV viremia or immunodeficiency. Even in patients with well-controlled HIV, there is an increased risk for diabetes, cancer, cardiovascular disease, osteoporosis, pulmonary disease, and more. Not only is there an increased risk of these conditions, but also it is suggested that these conditions may appear at earlier ages than would be expected in adults living without HIV. Healthcare systems and caregivers will have to adapt to the needs of this graying of the epidemic.

Studies have shown that geriatric syndromes, such as frailty, may also appear at younger ages in PLWH than in their matched peers. The manifestations of the syndromes will depend on myriad factors, including how many years they have lived with HIV and their biologic age, rather than their actual chronologic age. The picture is different for an older patient who acquires HIV now at 50 years old versus someone who is now 55 and has lived with the virus for over 25 years. While frailty is a natural consequence of old age, the earlier appearance in PLWH will take a toll on patients' livelihoods, ability to live independently, and to care for themselves. Providers are able to assess for frailty using a variety of assessment calculators, such as the Freid Index. This particular index will measure a patient's frailty based on weight loss, energy levels, physical activity, weakness, and walking speed. As important as it is to recognize these conditions, it is also important to note that this condition may be irreversible, and patients may not expect to return to their baseline level of functioning. Providers will need to identify support systems to assist in care for individuals during the aging process and attempt to slow the onset of geriatric conditions. In recent years, there has been increased interest in the physiological and genetic factors associated with aging, particularly in individuals living with HIV, and there is some research to suggest that exercise and physical activity can slow progression of frailty.

Menopause has also been suggested to have an accelerated timeline in women aging with HIV. Earlier onset of menopause may thereafter increase risk of osteoporosis and cardiovascular events—conditions for which elderly women with HIV may already be at risk. While a consistently undetectable viral load will improve long-term outcomes, it does not eliminate the risk of these consequences.

Substance abuse is yet another challenge providers can expect to face in this unique population. One study found that of PLWH over the age of 50, use of illicit drugs within the past year was reported by 48%. Furthermore, 73% had smoked cigarettes during their life, and 46% were current smokers—rates much higher than individuals of the same age without HIV. Substance use may contribute to difficulty managing medications, keeping appointments, and maintaining stable housing and can increase risk of malignancy, cardiovascular disease, and stroke, conditions that already present increased risks in PLWH. Smoking is the greatest risk factor for non-AIDS cancers in PLWH, and avoiding smoking could prevent up to one-third of these malignancies. Smoking cessation counseling at each visit and the use of medication therapy, including nicotine replacement therapies and others such as bupropion and Chantix, have had some positive results in this population.

Polypharmacy, defined as the simultaneous use of 5 or more medications, is another concern commonly seen in the elderly population, but especially in people aging with HIV (PAWH). Antiretroviral medications often have drug-drug interactions and cumulative adverse reactions. PAWH may have been on older antiretroviral medications with debilitating and chronic adverse reactions, such as lipodystrophy or nephrotoxicity. With neurocognitive disorders and depression, which may be subtle or undiagnosed, the potential morbidity and mortality from polypharmacy cannot be understated. Commonly used medications such as statins, beta-blockers, narcotics and analgesics, psychotropic drugs, and diuretics can potentially interact with HIV medications or lead to cognitive impairments, hypotension, and falls. Polypharmacy also increases the risk of poor adherence, thus increasing the risk for poor outcomes.

Finally, elderly PLWH often face loneliness, social isolation, and stigmata that can accelerate age-related conditions. The consequences of social isolation and loneliness cannot be understated in elderly PLWH. Many individuals have lost partners or friends to HIV. Others have been isolated from their families and communities due to stigmata. Rates of depression are greatly increased in PLWH and especially in elderly PLWH. These conditions affect not only a person's mental health, social isolation, and loneliness but also have been associated with a higher risk of cognitive decline, dementia, lowered immune function, obesity, and other health conditions. While addressing these issues may feel daunting, there is promise in offering elderly PLWH support services and treatment for mental health conditions.

As demonstrated, PAWH are at risk for numerous conditions that are further complicated by increased rates of loneliness, social isolation, substance abuse, frailty, and polypharmacy. These conditions are intertwined, synergistic, and accelerated by the aging process and HIV. Providers need to recognize the consequence of these conditions in order to properly care for elderly HIV-infected persons.

BACK TO OUR CASE

So, what is next for the patient described in this case? Her differential diagnosis remains broad as she has an increased risk for multiple conditions that could cause her symptoms. Malignancy—mainly breast, lung, and colon cancer—remains high on her differential. She is also at risk for AIDS-related lymphomas despite having well-controlled HIV. However, her symptoms could also be explained by less threatening conditions, such as hypothyroidism, anemia, menopause, vitamin deficiencies, or malnutrition. To evaluate potential etiologies, she will require laboratory assessment, imaging studies, appropriate cancer screenings, and referrals to specialists, such as ophthalmology. Change in vision could be caused by a relatively straightforward diagnoses, such as cataracts, or a more complex HIV-related diagnosis such as progressive outer retinal necrosis, though this is usually observed in patients with severely depressed immune systems.

Ordering basic laboratory tests and making referrals for specialists and screening tests is a logical place to start with this patient. Ruling out the organic diagnoses may actually be much simpler than addressing her frailty and decline in ability to perform activities of daily living (ADLs). Labs such as for vitamin B_{12}, Folate, MMA, thyroid-stimulating hormone, chemistry, complete cell count, and rapid plasma reagin (RPR) would be reasonable considering her complaints. She does not report muscle pain, but with her statin use and other unknown supplements, a check of her creatine kinase (CPK) to rule out a myopathy is warranted.

The Geriatric Assessment, Get Up and Go Test, or the Mini-Cog are relatively simple assessments that can be performed during a clinic visit and give providers a clearer understanding of her ability to perform ADLs. A Get Up and Go Test asks a patient to simply stand from a seating position without the use of arm rests, walk 10 feet, turn, and return to the chair. Those who have difficulty completing the task or take longer than 10 seconds to complete are noted to have an increased risk of falls. A Mini-Cog is a tool that can be completed in just a couple of minutes with a short series of written and spoken questions that assess a patient for signs of cognitive disorders or dementia. A complete neurocognitive assessment can begin with laboratory work and Mini-Mental State Examination, but may also require imagining to rule out white matter disease or space-occupying lesions. A referral to a neurologist may be necessary for a complete work up which may require additional testing. In some cases, a cerebrospinal fluid HIV viral load evaluation to rule a viral reservoir in the central nervous system will be indicated. Her CD4 count is over 500, and her risk of opportunistic infections is extremely low, but not impossible.

In addition, she is obese despite her recent weight loss. She should be counseled on calorie restriction and referred to a dietician if available to educate on a healthy diet. Furthermore, the role of exercise in maintaining muscle mass and preventing falls should be emphasized once she is evaluated for metabolic causes of her weakness. As described previously, exercise is shown be associated with slowing of the aging process.

Addressing her polypharmacy can be done in a primary care visit and may have almost immediate effects. One of the aspects of geriatric medicine is an evidence-based guide to de-prescribing or the supervised discontinuation of inappropriate medications. In this case, there are multiple medications that do not have clear indications. If she is not experiencing difficulty with sleep, trazodone may contribute to falls and fatigue. Addressing the indication for pantoprazole can prevent long-term adverse reactions and drug-drug interactions if she is to start hepatitis C therapy. Given that her blood pressure is low at today's visit, it may be reasonable to consider lowering the dose of the antihypertensive or discontinue her beta-blocker to prevent hypotension and falls. A review of her current and previous antiretrovirals can potentially help narrow to a single-tablet regimen and assess for adverse reactions of these medications. These are just a few examples of how consistent medication reconciliation is essential in the elderly population.

Finally, it is also essential to consider her social circumstances. She admits that she cannot reliably take her medications daily and does not have family at home to help her. She will also require assistance with transportation to multiple upcoming medical appointments. In cases such as this, a care coordinator or social worker can help identify available resources. Many insurance companies offer transportation to appointments. A social worker may also be able to assist in setting up home health care, such as having a certified nursing assistant visit biweekly. If these resources are unavailable or inadequate, a conversation about skilled nursing facilities may need to take place. Understandably so, many of these tasks cannot be performed at a single office visit. However, arranging appointments to address these issues would be reasonable. In the meantime, simpler solutions such organizing pillboxes can decrease the burden of multiple pill bottles. Many clinics also offer group therapy for patients such as this who would benefit from social support.

Health service integration will become increasingly important in aging patients. Collocation of primary, specialty, and psychosocial services is an approach that is needed. In settings where this is not possible, use of adjunctive telehealth may be beneficial. Using a systematic approach will help clinicians tackle one issue at a time. The 5 *M*s (mobility, mind, medications, multimorbidity, and what matters most) of geriatric care are increasingly pertinent to aging patients with HIV and should be addressed on a regular basis. Recognizing the most pertinent issue and addressing that first will keep appointments at an appropriate length.

> **KEY POINTS TO REMEMBER**
>
> · Elderly patients with HIV are at an increased risk for non–AIDs-related conditions, such as cancer, heart disease, osteoporosis, and kidney disease. They also may have an earlier onset of frailty and geriatric syndromes.
> · Resources in both the clinic and community settings are key. In the complex elderly PLWH, a multidisciplinary approach is needed to coordinate care.
> · Consider starting geriatric and frailty assessments in older PLWH at earlier ages than their peers not infected with HIV.
> · Incorporate the 5 *M*'s of geriatric care into the comprehensive care plan.

Further Reading

Brown B, Marg L, Cabral A. Community-driven health priorities for health aging with HIV. *J Assoc Nurses AIDs Care.* 2019;30(1):119–128.

Cahill S, Valadez R. Growing older with HIV/AIDS: new public health challenges. *Am J Public Health.* 2013;103(3):e7–e15. doi:10.2105/AJPH.2012.301161

Desquilbet L, Jacobson LP, Fried LP, et al. HIV-1 infection is associated with an earlier occurrence of a phenotype related to frailty. *J Gerontol A Biol Sci Med Sci.* 2007;62(11):1279–1286. doi:10.1093/gerona/62.11.1279

Greene M, Covinsky KE, Valcour V, et al. Geriatric syndromes in older HIV-infected adults. *J Acquir Immune Defic Syndr.* 2015;69(2):161–167. doi:10.1097/QAI.0000000000000556

Safreed-Harmon K, Anderson J, Azzopardi-Muscat N, et al. Reorienting health systems to care for people with HIV beyond viral suppression. *Lancet HIV.* 2019;e869–e877.

Sundermann EE, Erlandson KM, Pope CN, et al. Current challenges and solutions in research and clinic care of older persons living with HIV: findings presented at the 9th International Workshop on HIV and Aging. *AIDS Res Hum Retroviruses.* 2019;35(11–12):985–998. doi:10.1089/AID.2019.0100

Wing EJ. HIV and aging. *Int J Infect Dis.* 2016;53:61–68. doi:https://doi.org/10.1016/j.ijid.2016.10.004

20 "Is the bright red patch on the roof of my mouth related to the purple splotches on my back?"

Juliana Netto and Monica Merçon

A 35-year-old male newly diagnosed with HIV was referred to clinic complaining of numerous flat, violaceus skin lesions on his trunk and upper and lower limbs and a flat violaceus lesion on the palate, with early satiety.

His HIV viral load (VL) was 480,000 copies/mL with CD4+ 18 cells/mm^3 on antiretroviral therapy (ART) initiation with tenofovir/emtricitabine/elviltegravir/cobicistat. After a skin biopsy, the patient was discharged with trimethoprim-sulfamethoxazole for *Pneumocystis jiroveci* prophylaxis. Ten days after starting ART, he came to the emergency department with intense fatigue, fever, and difficulty swallowing. The lesion on the palate had become vegetating; skin lesions became larger and nodular, with bulky left cervical lymphadenomegaly. His heart rate was 120 beats per minute, and blood pressure was 90/60 mm Hg.

Laboratory results at admission showed HIV VL 840 copies/mL, CD4+ 70 cells/mm^3, hemoglobin 6.8 mg/dL, platelets 70,000 cells/mm^3, C-reactive protein (CRP) 6.5 mg/dL, albumin 2.6 mg/dL, and sodium 127 mEq/L.

What Do You Do Now?

KAPOSI SARCOMA WORSENING AFTER ART INTRODUCTION

After admission, esophagogastricduodenoscopy (EGD) showed lesions consistent with gastroduodenal Kaposi sarcoma (KS), and the skin biopsy result confirmed KS.

Kaposi sarcoma herpesvirus (KSHV), also known as HHV-8 (human herpesvirus 8), is the etiological agent of the following clinical conditions:

* Kaposi sarcoma
* Multicentric Castleman disease (MCD)
* Primary effusion lymphoma (PEL)
* KSHV inflammatory cytokine syndrome (KICS)

Unlike other herpesviruses, the prevalence of KSHV varies widely between different populations. In general, KSHV is highly prevalent in sub-Saharan Africa, is of intermediate prevalence in the Mediterranean and parts of South America, and has a low prevalence in the general population in northern Europe, North America, and Asia.

The transmission of KSHV varies in different populations. This virus can be secreted in saliva, and this is considered to be the main means of transmission. KSHV can eventually be transmitted by blood transfusion, but even in places with high seroprevalence, this risk is less than 3%.

After infection by KSHV, the genome is maintained in the nucleus of the host cells. KSHV can infect a variety of cell types, such as endothelial cells, B cells, and monocytes. After infection of a cell, KSHV goes into latency, during which there is expression of only a few genes, which help maintain the viral episome, escape the host's immune responses, and promote survival and proliferation of infected cells.

Some physiological signals lead the virus to enter the lytic phase, when all its genes are expressed, virions are produced and released, leading the infected cell to death. This transition from the latency phase to the lytic phase is triggered by a protein, the replication and transcription activator. In addition to physiological stressors, such as hypoxia, chemical agents such as valproic acid and sodium butyrate can induce the lytic cycle.

Transformation is a key event for the various stages of the oncogenesis process. It involves changes in signaling pathways and cell morphology, leading to a state of uncontrolled proliferation. Infection by KSHV of endothelial cells and/or hematopoietic progenitors leads to changes in their morphology, metabolism, growth rate, life span, and gene expression, resulting in KS. The oncogenicity of KSHV is reflected by the numerous pro-angiogenic molecules that are induced after infection of the endothelial cells. However, although KSHV has oncogenic genes that can potentially induce malignancy phenotypes, infection with this virus rarely leads to KS in the general population. This suggests that there are cofactors, such as HIV, that appear to have a direct role in KS oncogenesis or drug-induced immunosuppression and are necessary for the virus to induce the tumor.

Performing real-time polymerase chain reaction (PCR) for KSHV as a follow-up routine during KS treatment is expensive and laborious and is not indicated. However, although its value as a prognostic marker is controversial in the literature, the quantification of VL at the beginning of treatment may indicate to us the patients at greatest risk of developing severe forms of the disease. These are individuals who should be followed up with more frequent clinical reevaluations and also suggests when and for whom it is mandatory to perform imaging tests, such as computed tomography (CT), for the earlier detection of changes suggestive of other diseases related to KSHV, such as PEL, MCD, and KICS, which may have a more aggressive clinical course.

Kaposi sarcoma is the most common neoplasm in patients with acquired immunodeficiency syndrome (AIDS) and is responsible for significant morbidity and mortality. Although the incidence of AIDS-associated KS has declined since the implementation of combination ART, it remains a major clinical problem.

This patient presented with advanced immunodeficiency on HIV diagnosis with a CD4+ cell count of 18 cells/mm^3. An initial low CD4 cell count and rapid decline of plasma HIV VL are major risk factors for immune reconstitution inflammatory syndrome (IRIS). Worsening of symptoms, including enlargement of skin and palate lesions, just after starting ART may be attributable to KS-IRIS. There is evidence suggesting that integrase strand transfer inhibitors (INSTIs), such as elvitegravir in this case, may be associated with a higher risk for IRIS. Nodular, violaceus skin lesions and vegetating oral lesions are shown in Figure 20.1.

The typical recovery of CD4+ lymphocytes after the onset of ART is biphasic. A rapid increase in the count of these lymphocytes occurs during

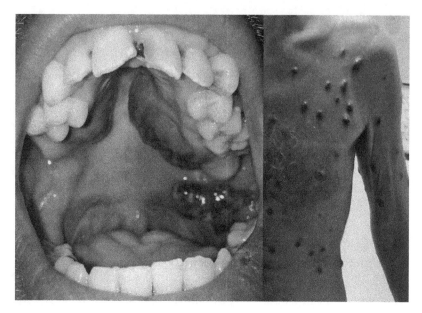

FIGURE 20.1 Vegetating oral lesions and nodular, violaceus skin lesions.

the first 6 months of ART. This initial recovery is mainly due to an increase in memory T cells, combined with a decrease in lymphocyte apoptosis and lymphocyte redistribution of peripheral lymphoid tissues into the bloodstream. Then, there is a slight increase in naïve CD4+ lymphocytes in most patients, believed to be an expansion of T-cell clones produced in the thymus. Concomitantly, there is a rapid increase in CD8+ lymphocytes after the initiation of ART. In vitro studies showed that there is an important increase in the production of immune activation and delayed hypersensitivity markers.

As the onset of ART leads to a rapid increase in CD4+ lymphocytes in peripheral blood in most patients, some studies have shown that there is an increase in T helper type 1 (Th1) response to antigens after installation of ART. A deregulation of the control of the inflammatory response may also be associated with IRIS. Studies showed that there is a decrease in the number of regulatory lymphocytes and interleukin (IL) 10 in patients with IRIS, and that the involvement of the innate immune response plays an important role in the pro-inflammatory development of these patients.

Kaposi sarcoma–associated IRIS occurs in 7%–31% of cases, and this variation may be related to the severity of KS, degree of immunosuppression, and the availability of specific treatment in different locations. There is an increased risk of IRIS when using ART alone as an initial therapy for KS. More advanced tumor staging, HIV initial VL above 100,000 copies/mL, and detectable KSHV VL in plasma at the onset of ART are also risk factors associated with KS-related IRIS. The temporal relationship between the initiation of ART for HIV and the appearance of manifestations related to the inflammatory response is also an important factor for the diagnostic hypothesis of IRIS. Mean time between the initiation of ART and the development of IRIS is 48 days, but it can occur up to 6 months after the initiation of ART.

IMMUNE RECONSTITUTION SYNDROME AND KAPOSI SARCOMA

Criteria for the Diagnosis of IRIS

The following are KS exacerbation criteria for IRIS diagnosis:

Sudden increase in number and/or size of lesions up to 6 months after ART initiation.
Involvement of previously disease-free sites.
Emergence or exacerbation of lymphedema.

The following are laboratory criteria for IRIS diagnosis:

At least 1 $\log^{10}$ reduction in HIV VL and/or CD4 count greater or equal to 50 cells/mm^3 within 6 months of ART onset.
Other reasons for worsening KS must be discarded (e.g., the predictable evolution of the clinical course of the disease, chemotherapy withdrawal, suspension of ART).

Treatment of KS-Associated IRIS

Corticosteroids are contraindicated in KS-IRIS since they may further exacerbate KS lesions due to the synergy of cytokines with glucocorticoid receptors in KS spindle cells. KSHV-specific immune reconstitution and the antiviral effect of combined ART plus chemotherapy have been recently documented, with a trend toward better clinical outcome compared to ART alone. In some situations, a temporary withdrawal from ART may be desirable, with reintroduction after control of inflammatory manifestations.

In a severely immunodeficient patient with lymphadenopathy, hematological abnormalities and fever are relatively common and should be investigated within a broad framework. In general, disseminated endemic mycosis, like *Histoplasma capsulatum*; *Cryptococcus* spp; *Mycobacterium* spp, mainly tuberculosis; visceral leishimaniasis where the disease is endemic; bacteria-like *Bartonella henselae*, which can cause violaceus lesions very similar to KS; and malignancies should be included in the differential diagnosis. Complete investigation for infection must be performed, including investigation of blood, urine, sputum, and a lymph node biopsy since they are key for the diagnosis. Among malignancies that can cause these symptoms, non-Hodgkin lymphoma (the most common type of lymphoma in patients living with HIV/AIDS) and visceral KS are the most frequent. More specifically, in this case, as the patient has diffuse KS lesions, all the systemic manifestations may be caused by KS itself or another KSHV-associated malignancy.

The differential diagnosis is made exclusively by lymph node biopsy, and it is possible that the biopsy can reveal the association of KS and MCD, for example. KS-positive lymph nodes show tumor infiltration, which may be may be uni- or multifocal, and the lymph node may be entirely affected. The alterations consist of spindle cells, a proliferation of abnormal vessels, and increased permeability, with overflow of blood cells and hemosiderin deposits, with prominent inflammatory infiltrate. Immunohistochemistry for KSHV is routinely performed and confirms the diagnosis. There is no histopathological difference between KS and KS-associated IRIS.

A CT scan of the patient's chest showed bilateral pleural effusion, minimal pericardial effusion (Figure 20.2), and peribronchovascular infiltrates. A peribronchovascular infiltrate is characteristic of KS pulmonary involvement. Pleural effusions can be caused by any of the KSHV-associated diseases. If possible, thoracentesis with pleural biopsy for histopathological examination with immunohistochemistry for KSHV should be performed. The hypothesis of PEL should be considered whenever a patient living with

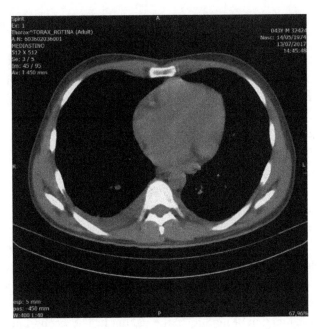

FIGURE 20.2 Computed tomographic scan with bilateral pleural and pericardial effusions.

HIV/AIDS presents with cavity effusions, especially those with KS and/or inflammatory symptoms, similar to MCD and KICS. Even small effusions should be considered.

Kaposi sarcoma herpesvirus inflammatory cytokine syndrome was described in 2010 by Uldrick et al. following the observation of several patients living with HIV with KS or serological evidence of KSHV infection who had significant inflammatory symptoms similar to MCD but in whom MCD could not be diagnosed. Thus, KICS should be included in the differential diagnosis of diffuse lymphadenopathy with severe inflammatory symptoms, although it may occur in the absence of lymphadenomegaly. This patient had laboratory abnormalities such as anemia, thrombocytopenia, hypoalbuminemia, and hyponatremia. Also, the patient had respiratory abnormalities (peribronchovascular infiltrates); body cavity effusion (bilateral pleural effusion); gastrointestinal (GI) symptoms (postprandial plenitude); fever and fatigue; and elevated CRP. It is essential to collect a blood sample to measure the KSHV VL since detectable KSHV plasma VL above 1000 copies/mL or peripheral blood mononuclear cells (PBMCs) above 100 copies/10^6 cells is a criteria for KICS diagnosis. The patient's KSHV plasma VL was 3.6×10^3 copies/mL.

This patient had disseminated KS disease with extensive skin, oral, pulmonary, and gastric involvement. Lymph node and pleural biopsy were positive for KS. Once the diagnosis was confirmed by biopsy, and considering the severity of the clinical presentation, specific chemotherapy must be started.

The first-line chemotherapy regimen for KS is liposomal doxorubicin, an anthracycline. Advantages of using liposomal doxorubicin include a longer plasma half-life, a high tumor concentration of the drug, and less toxicity to nontarget organs. Compared to other regimens with nonliposomal anthracyclines, the toxicity of liposomal anthracyclines occurs substantially less frequently. Hair loss is rare, and the incidence of cardiac toxicity, even after high accumulated doses, seems to be quite low. Even with reduced cardiotoxicity in relation to other regimens, it is recommended that an echocardiogram be performed before starting the treatment, and that cardiac function be monitored throughout it. The second-line regimen is paclitaxel (PTX), a drug with proven efficacy, even for anthracycline-resistant KS. PTX may be associated with alopecia, myalgia, arthralgia, and myelosuppression. Although adverse events such as neutropenia and alopecia are more frequent with PTX, taking into account the good response rate and much lower cost, the treatment with this chemotherapy is a cost-effective option in low-income countries. Due to the multiple toxicities associated with these drugs, KS treatment must be conducted by an experienced professional.

Since MCD and PEL were excluded by lymph node and pleural biopsies, we concluded the patient's diagnosis was KS and KICS. It is also unclear how to best treat this condition. The most recommended approach would be to treat the underlying tumors and to explore treatment options that were developed for KSHV-MCD, such as rituximab.

A SUMMARY OF KSHV-ASSOCIATED DISEASES

Kaposi Sarcoma

Kaposi sarcoma most often comes in the form of violaceus skin lesions. Lymph nodes are the second most common site of involvement by the disease, followed by the GI tract and respiratory tract. GI involvement is usually asymptomatic, not affecting prognosis.

Skin lesions appear most frequently on the lower extremities, face (particularly on the tip of the nose), and genitals. They are usually pigmented, ranging from pink to violet, or brown in color. Skin lesions are often multifocal, and the lower limbs and soles of the feet may form plaques or have a fungoid appearance. The lesions may become ulcerated. Lymphatic edema, particularly on the face, genitalia, and lower limbs, may be extensive. Oral cavity involvement is common, occurs in about 33% of cases, and may be the initial site of the disease. In the head and neck, any location can be affected, including the salivary glands and larynx, where it can cause airway obstruction. Visceral involvement occurs in more than 50% of cases, although only a few become symptomatic. GI involvement was described at initial diagnosis in 40% of cases and up to 80% of autopsies.

The clinical course is variable, ranging from a slow, indolent process requiring little or no treatment to a rapidly progressive and fatal disease. While many patients progress well only with the introduction of ART, others have a progressive disease that requires chemotherapy. In addition, as mentioned, KS can be further complicated by IRIS and KICS.

SYMPTOMS AND SIGNS OF KICS

Symptoms of KICS are fever, fatigue, edema, cachexia, respiratory symptoms, GI disorders, arthralgia, and myalgia. Also included are alteration of mental state and neuropathy with or without pain.

Laboratory changes associated with KICS are anemia, thrombocytopenia, hypoalbuminemia, and hyponatremia.

The KICS radiological changes can involve lymphadenopathy, splenomegaly, hepatomegaly, and body cavity effusions.

Elevated CRP is evidence of systemic inflammation.

Evidence of KSHV Viral Activity

The KSHV viral plasma load is above 1000 cps/mL or PBMCs above 100 copies/10^6 cells.

The absence of KSHV-associated MCD is diagnostically excluded by biopsy. In the differential diagnosis for KICS are MCD and PEL, but infection must always be ruled out.

It is also unclear how to best treat this condition. Treating the underlying tumors and exploring approaches developed for KSHV-MCD are considered.

Next is a brief description of MCD and PEL clinical presentations.

MULTICENTRIC CASTLEMAN DISEASE

Multicentric Castleman disease is a lymphoproliferative disease characterized by recurrent episodes of fever, generalized lymphadenopathy, hepatosplenomegaly, anemia, thrombocytopenia, hypoalbuminemia, hyponatremia, polyclonal hypergammaglobulinemia, and elevated inflammatory markers such as CRP. Very intense inflammatory symptoms, which can mimic sepsis, can confuse the clinician, delaying the diagnosis and negatively affecting the prognosis of this potentially fatal condition.

The histopathological diagnosis of MCD is usually based on an excisional lymph node biopsy, showing expansion of reactive plasma cells, interspersed with KSHV-infected plasmablasts, as well as hyalinization of lymphoid follicles and increased hair proliferation. A significant part of these cells express Viral interleukin 6 (vIL-6), and a smaller number also express other lytic antigens of KSHV. In addition to the propensity to develop tumors, MCD in individuals living with HIV is a more aggressive disease than in individuals not infected with HIV. Without treatment, KSHV-MCD is generally lethal. Before specific therapies were developed, observed overall survival was 2 years or less. Rituximab, a monoclonal anti-CD20 antigen, dramatically improved the prognosis of patients with this clinical condition, and a combination of rituximab and cytotoxic chemotherapy is recommended, as rituximab can lead to worsening KS.

PRIMARY EFFUSION LYMPHOMA

Primary effusion lymphoma is a KSHV-associated neoplasm that involves the pleural, pericardial, or peritoneal cavities without forming a mass. It is a rare, aggressive, B-cell neoplasm that accounts for 1% to 4% of

HIV-associated lymphomas and less than 1% of non–HIV-associated lymphomas. It is a monoclonal B-cell lymphoma associated with KSHV, most common in patients living with HIV/AIDS, that has a poor prognosis. Extracavitary PEL refers to a solid tumor that has characteristics similar to conventional PEL.

Most patients who develop PEL have immunosuppression and, in the United States, most patients with PEL are adult men living with HIV. The median patient age is about 45 years. Up to two-thirds of patients with PEL concurrently or previously have had KS, and about one-third have had Castleman disease. PEL can develop in patients not living with HIV, including in the posttransplant setting. Rare patients with PEL do not have a history or evidence of immunosuppression.

Historically, median survival was less than 6 months. Nonetheless, PEL should be approached with curative intent. Combination therapy with a regimen based on CHOP (cyclophosphamide, doxorubicin, vincristine, and prednisone) and combination ART is commonly used as first-line therapy and may lead to long-term remissions in approximately 40% of patients. Although relatively rare, it is probably underdiagnosed.

Clinical Presentation

- Lymphomatous cavity effusions, most often pleural, may also affect pericardium, cause ascites, or even affect joints.
- Extracavitary forms may affect the skin, lymph nodes, GI tract, and central nervous system.

KEY POINTS TO REMEMBER

- Kaposi sarcoma is the most common neoplasm in patients living with HIV/AIDS.
- Kaposi sarcoma herpesvirus, also known as HHV-8, is the etiological agent of KS, MCD, PEL, and KICS.
- Kaposi sarcoma–associated IRIS can lead to worsening of preexistent KS lesions, as well as lead to the emergence of new ones, and can be a severe clinical condition.

- Liposomal doxorubicin is considered the first-line regimen for KS. PTX is a drug with proven efficacy, even for anthracycline-resistant KS, and is considered the second-line treatment.
- In a setting of a severely immunodeficient patient with a diagnosis of KS, lymphadenopathy, hematological abnormalities, and fever, it is important to investigate within a broad framework, including infectious diseases, other KSHV-associated conditions, and lymphoproliferative disorders.

Further Reading

Dutertre M, Cuzin L, Demonchy E, et al. Initiation of antiretroviral therapy containing integrase inhibitors increases the risk of iris requiring hospitalization. *J Acquir Immune Defic Syndr*. 2017;76(1):e23–e26.

Goncalves PH, Zielgelbauer J, Uldrick TS, Yarchoan R. Kaposi sarcoma herpesvirus-associated cancers and related diseases. *Curr Opin HIV AIDS*. 2017;12(1):47–56.

Haddow LJ, Easterbrook PJ, Mosam A, et al. Defining immune reconstitution inflammatory syndrome: evaluation of expert opinion versus 2 case definitions in a South African cohort. *Clin Infect Dis*. 2009;49(9):1424–1432.

Ingeborg Wijting CR, Wit F, Postma A, et al. Integrase inhibitors are an independent risk factor for iris: an ATHENA cohort study. Poster presented at *CROI*. February 13–17, 2017; Seattle, WA.

Letang E, Lewis JJ, Bower M, et al. Immune reconstitution inflammatory syndrome associated with Kaposi sarcoma: higher incidence and mortality in Africa than in the UK. *AIDS*. 2013;27(10):1603–1613.

Lilly AJ, Fedoriw Y. Human immunodeficiency virus-associated lymphoproliferative disorders. *Surg Pathol*. 2019;12:771–782.

Polizzotto MN, Uldrick TS, Wyvill KM, et al. Clinical features and outcomes of patients with symptomatic Kaposi sarcoma herpesvirus (KSHV)-associated inflammation: prospective characterization of KSHV inflammatory cytokine syndrome (KICS). *Clin Infect Dis*. 2016;62(6):730–738.

Sukswai N, Lyapichev K, Khoury JD, Medeiros LJ, Diffuse large B-cell lymphoma variants: an update. *Pathology*. 2020;52(1):P53–P67. https://doi.org/10.1016/j.pathol.2019.08.013

Uldrick TS, Wang V, O'Mahony D, et al. An interleukin-6-related systemic inflammatory syndrome in patients co-infected with Kaposi sarcoma-associated herpesvirus and HIV but without multicentric Castleman disease. *Clin Infect Dis*. 2010;51(3):350–358.

Walker NF, Scriven J, Meintjes G, Wilkinson R. Immune reconstitution inflammatory syndrome in HIV-infected patients. *HIV/AIDS (Auckl)*. 2015;7:49–64.

21 "I feel fine. Do I really need to take a cholesterol pill?"

Arvind Nishtala and Matthew J. Feinstein

Mr. Brown is a 57-year-old African American male who's close friend just died of a major heart attack, and he is concerned about his own risk. He has no hypertension or diabetes. He quit smoking in 2000, has not used any illicit substances since 2000, and he only drinks an occasional glass of wine on holidays. He has no family history of cardiovascular disease (CVD). His blood pressure is 124/76 mm Hg and body mass index is 27.3. His total cholesterol is 180 mg/dL, high-density lipoprotein cholesterol (HDL-C) is 55 mg/dL, triglycerides are 75 mg/dL, and low-density lipoprotein cholesterol (LDL-C) is 110 mg/dL. His hemoglobin A_1 is 5.8. He does not have hepatitis C virus. He was diagnosed with HIV in 1994 when treated for *Pneumocystis jiroveci* pneumonia. He had a period of uncontrolled viremia and a nadir CD4 count of 78 cells/mm³. He has since been virally suppressed with incomplete immunologic recovery, with CD4 counts in the 300–500 range over the past 10 years (most recently 372). His only medications are dolutegravir and tenofovir alafenamide/emtricitabine.

What Do You Do Now?

HIV AND CARDIOVASCULAR DISEASE

HIV has transformed into a manageable chronic disease in many settings because of the effectiveness and widespread uptake of combination antiretroviral therapy (ART). People with HIV (PWH) are living longer than previously but experience chronic inflammation and immune dysregulation, treatment toxicity, morbidity unrelated to HIV infection and acquired immune deficiency syndrome (AIDS), and geriatric syndromes.

People with HIV are specifically experiencing a high burden of CVDs and are at greater risk of CVD than uninfected individuals. Although the use of effective ART has decreased the relative risk of cardiovascular complications, the overall burden of HIV-associated CVD tripled over the past two decades. PWH face an approximately 1.5-fold increased risk of atherosclerotic CVD (ASCVD), including myocardial infarction (MI) and stroke, and heart failure (HF) compared with persons not infected with HIV. This remains true among PWH with viral suppression, although lower CD4 counts and higher levels of viremia are associated with increased relative risks of MI, stroke, and HF.

PATHOPHYSIOLOGY OF ASCVD AND HF IN PLWH

The underlying pathophysiologic processes that drive the increased risk of CVD in PWH are still not completely understood and are under active study. Several studies have clarified contributions and coaction of traditional cardiovascular risk factors, chronic inflammation and immune dysregulation, and off-target effects of certain antiretrovirals.

Traditional ASCVD Risk Factors. PWH have a high prevalence of traditional cardiovascular risk factors. HIV infection is associated with metabolic derangements, including dyslipidemia and insulin resistance, which in turn can lead to CVD. The dyslipidemia in HIV is thought to be characterized by elevated triglyceride levels without an elevation of LDL-C. Hypertriglyceridemia was initially a consequence of specific early ART medications, including protease inhibitors (PIs) and efavirenz, but the contemporary ART regimens have minimal lipid effects. Despite the lack of LDL-C elevation, dyslipidemia in HIV is atherogenic and an independent risk factor for atherosclerotic CVD. Insulin resistance and diabetes mellitus are common in persons living with HIV (PLWH) and contribute to a greater than 2-fold increase in risk for atherosclerotic CVD events in these individuals. In addition to hypertension, dyslipidemia, and insulin resistance, there are high rates of smoking, heavy alcohol use, and other substance use that contribute to a greater risk of CVD.

Chronic Inflammation and Immune Dysregulation. Even after adjustment for traditional CVD risk factors (including smoking), several studies in large cohorts demonstrated heightened risks for MI, stroke, and HF among PWH. Chronic HIV-associated inflammation and immune dysregulation, even in the presence of effective viral control and CD4 recovery, are associated with and predictive of CVD and mortality overall, as well as subclinical measures of CVD. Although effective treatment with ART leading to viral suppression can decrease HIV-associated inflammation and CVD risk, it does not normalize these to levels comparable to individuals not infected with HIV.

The Role of ART. Since the landmark Strategic Timing of Antiretroviral Treatment (START) and Strategies for Management of Anti-Retroviral Therapy (SMART) trials, it has become clear that early and uninterrupted ART is essential for optimizing HIV control as well as limiting off-target comorbidities (including CVD). Nevertheless, certain ART medications have been associated with heightened relative risks for CVD and CVD risk factors. Several PIs, particularly older generation PIs with the exception of atazanavir, have been associated with an increased risk of MI as a class effect. Abacavir, a non-nucleoside reverse transcriptase inhibitor (NRTI), has been associated with an increased risk of MI and with worse outcomes following HF onset, although not all analyses of abacavir found this as a consistent effect. More recently, concerns related to integrase inhibitor–associated weight gain have come to the forefront; while the impact of this on hard clinical endpoints remains to be seen, PWH with high cardiometabolic risks who could be adversely affected by weight gain may need to be followed particularly closely for CVD (including HF) development if started on integrase inhibitors.

CVD RISK ASSESSMENT IN PWH

Estimating a patient's overall CVD (and specifically ASCVD) risk is an important exercise to undertake because it allows patients and providers to obtain a general sense of the absolute risk for events and the resulting net clinical benefit (which weighs absolute risks against absolute benefit) of preventive interventions. The estimation of an individual's CVD risk allows the clinician to match the intensity of preventive efforts with the patient's risk, thereby maximizing anticipated benefit and minimizing potential harm from treatment. The toolkit for CVD risk assessment is derived from the American College of Cardiology/American Heart Association (ACC/AHA) guidelines on CVD risk assessment, lipid-lowering therapy, and primary prevention of CVD.

Traditional CVD and ASCVD risk estimators tend to underestimate risk for PWH. The ACC/AHA ASCVD Risk Estimator (https://tools.acc.org/ASCVD-Risk-Estimator-Plus/) incorporates the use of traditional cardiovascular risk factors, race, and sex and is used to estimate 10-year ASCVD risk in asymptomatic adults between 40 and 75 years of age using the Pooled Cohort Equations (PCE). Adults are classified as being low (<5%), borderline (5% to < 7.5%), intermediate (≥7.5% to < 20%), or high (≥20%) risk. While this calculator and others consistently underestimate CVD risk in PWH, they represent a useful starting point for clinician use to identify the contributions of traditional risk factors to a patient's expected ASCVD risk, understanding predicted risk levels represent the low-end range of the true risk for PWH.

As previously mentioned, HIV infection is an independent risk factor for CVD in addition to traditional cardiovascular risk factors. HIV-related factors that further enhance risk for CVD include any of the following (discussed in detail in the recent AHA Scientific Statement on HIV and CVD):

- History of prolonged viremia and/or delay in ART initiation
- Low current or nadir CD4 count (≥350 cells/mm³)
- HIV treatment failure or nonadherence
- Metabolic syndrome, HIV lipodystrophy, fatty liver disease
- Hepatitis C virus co-infection

Traditional risk-enhancing factors that increase individual ASCD risk have been well described in the ACC/AHA guidelines and include the following:

- Family history of premature ASCVD (males, age < 55 years; females, age < 65 years)

- Primary hypercholesterolemia (LDL-C, 160–189 mg/dL [4.1–4.8 mmol/L]; non–HDL-C 190–219 mg/dL [4.9–5.6 mmol/L])*
- Metabolic syndrome (increased waist circumference [by ethnically appropriate cut points], elevated triglycerides [>150 mg/dL, nonfasting], elevated blood pressure, elevated glucose, and low HDL-C [<40 mg/dL in men; < 50 mg/dL in women] are factors; a tally of 3 makes the diagnosis)
- Chronic kidney disease (estimated glomerular filtration rate 15–59 mL/min/1.73 m² with or without albuminuria; not treated with dialysis or kidney transplantation)
- Chronic inflammatory conditions, such as psoriasis, rheumatoid arthritis, or lupus
- History of premature menopause (before age 40 years) and history of pregnancy-associated conditions that increase later ASCVD risk, such as preeclampsia
- High-risk race/ethnicity (e.g., South Asian ancestry)
- Lipids/biomarkers associated with increased ASCVD risk (other than ones mentioned previously):
  - If measured:
    - Elevated high-sensitivity C-reactive protein (≥2.0 mg/L)
    - Elevated lipoprotein a [Lp(a)]. An Lp(a) 50 mg/dL or greater or 125 nmol/L or greater constitutes a risk-enhancing factor, especially at higher levels of Lp(a).
    - Elevated apolipoprotein B (apoB) (≥130 mg/dL). A level of 130 mg/dL or greater corresponds to an LDL-C greater than 160 mg/dL and constitutes a risk-enhancing factor.
    - Ankle-brachial index (<0.9).

In addition to these factors, the presence of subclinical atherosclerosis on imaging, such as the measurement of coronary artery calcium (CAC), is also used to reclassify risk upward. While those PWH with elevated CAC can be presumed to be at higher risk, the ability of CAC scoring to discriminate ASCVD risk in PLWH has not yet been determined. There are insufficient data currently to recommend routine measurement of subclinical atherosclerosis on imaging or inflammatory biomarkers because the additive value of these measurements for CVD risk stratification in HIV is unclear. Nevertheless, if already measured, atherosclerosis on imaging and elevated levels of Lp(a), high-sensitivity C-reactive protein, or apoB suggest higher ASCVD risk and may warrant more aggressive strategies for ASCVD prevention.

PRIMARY PREVENTION OF CVD IN PWH

As detailed in the 2019 ACC/AHA Guideline on the Primary Prevention of Cardiovascular Disease, the foundation of primary prevention of CVD in all individuals is the promotion of a healthy lifestyle across the life span.

All adults should be counseled on consuming a healthy diet that promotes the intake of vegetables, fruits, nuts, whole grains, lean vegetable or animal protein, and fish and minimizes the intake of trans fats, red meats, refined carbohydrates, and sweetened beverages. Overweight and obese individuals should be counseled on caloric restriction and the intake of nutrient-rich calories to achieve a healthy weight goal. All adults should partake in at least 150 minutes of moderate-intensity or 75 minutes of high-intensity physical activity weekly. There is evidence for improvement in systemic inflammation and cardiometabolic health with increasing physical activity among PLWH. There are resources online (https://www.HIV.gov and https://aids.nlm.nih.gov/topic/1141/living-with-hiv-aids/1146/) concerning exercise and physical fitness that cater to PLWH and that physicians will find useful when counseling their patients.

Smoking cessation is of utmost importance in reducing CVD risk, particularly given its increased prevalence among PLWH. In addition, physicians should be attentive to the increased prevalence of substance use and abuse in this population and screen and counsel appropriately. While there is no optimal dose of alcohol intake that has been determined, physicians should recommend that their patients consume fewer than 7 drinks weekly as the adverse effects of heavy alcohol use on CVD outcomes are well known.

The approach to treatment of hypertension or type 2 diabetes mellitus does not differ from the general population and should be focused on nonpharmacologic interventions prior to initiation of pharmacologic therapy. The recent emergence of evidence on use of glucagon-like peptide 1 agonists and sodium-glucose transport protein inhibitors for reduction of CVD events in the general population has not been extended to those with HIV, and these agents are not specifically recommended in the HIV population presently.

Statins play a central role in CVD risk reduction in the general population, and this benefit is thought to extend to those with HIV. PLWH often have normal LDL-C levels but increased systemic and arterial inflammation despite remaining virally suppressed with preserved CD4 counts on ART. When deciding on statin therapy, close attention needs to be paid to the patient's ART regimen due to drug-drug interactions as a result of cytochrome P450 (CYP) modulation. Simvastatin and lovastatin should be avoided in PLWH because they are extensively metabolized by the CYP system, which in turn is affected by ART medications. Pravastatin and pitavastatin are minimally metabolized by the CYP system and can be used without issue alongside ART regimens. Additionally, high-intensity statins such as atorvastatin and rosuvastatin can also be prescribed at their common doses without concern for significant CYP metabolism. While there is presently no robust data for statin use in primary prevention of CVD in PLWH, the ongoing Randomized Trial to Prevent Vascular Events in HIV (REPRIEVE) trial is studying the effect of pitavastatin on preventing CVD events in low- and moderate-risk patients and will offer a stronger evidence base for clinical decision-making in this realm. In the meantime, statin therapy should be offered for those with clinical ASCVD, LDL-C of greater than or equal to 190 mg/dL, and PLWH between the ages of 40–75 years old with comorbid diabetes. Additionally, following a thorough CVD risk assessment (as detailed in the previous section), statin therapy should be initiated in those deemed to be at sufficiently high CVD risk following a clinician-patient risk discussion (Figure 21.1).

The role of nonstatin lipid-lowering therapies, specifically the use of proprotein convertase subtilsin-kexin type 9 (PCSK9) inhibitors is not well known in the HIV population, and future studies are needed. Similarly, the role of anti-inflammatory therapies in PLWH to decrease CVD risk needs further study.

There is a dearth of evidence on the role that aspirin plays in primary prevention in PWH, but there are not enough data to offer a recommendation that is tailored to this population.

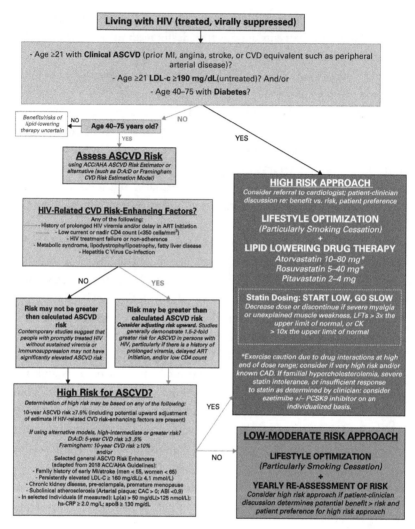

FIGURE 21.1 In the case of patient JB, the clinical decision pathway is highlighted by the boxes and grey arrows. A risk discussion between the clinician and patient is emphasized in order to determine whether lifestyle optimization and reassessment of risk or statin therapy are the chosen strategy. CAD, coronary artery disease. Adapted from AHA Scientific Statement on Characteristics, Prevention, and Management of Cardiovascular Disease in People Living with HIV.

BACK TO OUR CASE

Based on the ACC/AHA ASCVD Risk Estimator using the PCE, Mr. Brown's 10-year risk for an atherosclerotic CVD event is 6.5%. This is in the intermediate range (5%–7.4%), for which the guidelines in the general population recommend a risk discussion between the patient and clinician about initiating statin therapy after a thorough evaluation for risk-enhancing factors that may favor statin initiation is completed.

Mr. Brown does not have any traditional risk-enhancing factors that increase his CVD risk. However, he does carry a history of prolonged HIV viremia with delay in ART initiation and a low nadir (and somewhat low current) CD4 count, which may increase his 10-year risk of an atherosclerotic CVD event beyond that which was calculated using the PCE.

Therefore, the presence of HIV-related CVD risk-enhancing factors likely increase Mr. Brown's risk of an atherosclerotic CVD event such that statin therapy initiation is favored. In addition to initiation of statin therapy, preferably with atorvastatin, rosuvastatin, or pitavastatin, extensive counseling regarding lifestyle optimization with increasing levels of physical activity and healthy dietary consumption is recommended.

The risk calculus changes if we modify certain aspects of the case. Women living with HIV may actually carry a higher risk of MI and HF than their uninfected counterparts as well as men with HIV. Therefore, one may consider having a lower threshold for statin initiation in women living with HIV who carry a similar risk profile as their male counterparts. On the other hand, if a patient with a similar risk profile as Mr. Brown but with prompt initiation of ART after diagnosis, no sustained viremia, and no significant decline in CD4 count presented, the person's relative contribution of HIV-related risk-enhancing factors to overall CVD risk may be considerably less, and actual risk for ASCVD may be relatively similar to the predicted 6%–7%. In this case, a thorough discussion of risks and benefits of statin therapy, particularly in the setting of polypharmacy, would be warranted as this represents a true gray area of the net clinical benefit of lipid-lowering therapy.

- The transition of HIV to a chronic disease has increased the global burden of CVD among PWH.
- Persons with HIV have an increased risk of CVD compared to uninfected individuals, and their risk remains elevated despite being on effective ART with viral suppression and immunologic recovery.
- The pathophysiology of CVD risk among PWH is multifactorial and related to an increased burden of traditional cardiovascular risk factors, exposure to ART, and chronic inflammation and immune dysregulation.
- Precise CVD risk assessment in PWH is challenging. The approach to CVD risk assessment in PWH is based on the 2013 and 2018 ACC/AHA guidelines on CVD risk assessment and lipid-lowering therapy with the supplementation of specific HIV-related CVD risk-enhancing factors to modify the risk estimates derived from clinical risk-scoring calculators such as the PCE.
- The cornerstone of CVD prevention is lifestyle optimization and the promotion of healthy behaviors across the life span. Statin therapy is recommended for those deemed to be at high risk for a CVD event. The role of aspirin for primary prevention in PLWH is not clearly established.
- The AHA Scientific Statement on Characteristics, Prevention, and Management of Cardiovascular Disease in People Living With HIV published in 2019 is a valuable resource for better understanding the relationship between HIV and CVD.

Further Reading

Feinstein MJ, Hsue PY, Benjamin LA, et al. Characteristics, prevention, and management of cardiovascular disease in people living with HIV: a scientific statement from the American Heart Association. *Circulation*. 2019;140:e98–e124. doi:10.1161/cir.0000000000000695

Arnett DK, Blumenthal RS, Albert MA, et al. 2019 ACC/AHA guideline on the primary prevention of cardiovascular disease: a report of the American College of Cardiology/American Heart Association Task Force on Clinical Practice Guidelines.

Circulation. 2019;140:e596–e646. Originally published 17 March 2019. https://doi.
org/10.1161/CIR.0000000000000678

Grundy SM, Stone NJ, Bailey AL, et al. 2018 AHA/ACC/AACVPR/AAPA/ABC/
ACPM/ADA/AGS/APhA/ASPC/NLA/PCNA guideline on the management of
blood cholesterol: a report of the American College of Cardiology/American
Heart Association Task Force on Clinical Practice Guidelines. *Circulation.*
2019;139:e1082–e1143. Originally published 10 November 2018. https://doi.org/
10.1161/CIR.0000000000000625

"Am I going to need dialysis the rest of my life?"

Huma Saeed and Carlos A. Q. Santos

A 35-year-old male presents to clinic for evaluation. His medical history consists of HIV diagnosed 7 years ago through men who have sex with men (MSM) sexual contact. He was previously on abacavir, lamivudine, and dolutegravir, but was subsequently switched to tenofovir disoproxil fumarate weekly, lamivudine, and dolutegravir after developing a rash from abacavir. He reports excellent adherence with his new antiretroviral therapy (ART) regimen and remains virologically suppressed with a CD4 count of 488 checked 2 months prior. He is asymptomatic with no history of opportunistic infections. Other medical problems include hypertension and end-stage renal disease (ESRD) from immunoglobulin (Ig) A nephropathy. He was started on peritoneal dialysis 2 years ago and tolerates it well. Other medications include amlodipine, losartan, and atorvastatin. He is currently in a monogamous relationship with a person living with HIV (PLWH) and runs his own real estate agency. He denies any cigarette smoking or drug use. The examination today is unremarkable.

What Do You Do Now?

RENAL TRANSPLANT IN PERSONS LIVING WITH HIV

With the advent of highly efficacious ART regimens, individuals with HIV remain at increased risk for ESRD, mainly secondary to HIV-associated nephropathy, hepatitis-associated glomerulonephritis, membranous nephropathy, IgA nephropathy, and drug-related nephrotoxicity. As a result, renal transplant has become more common in PLWH and offers a survival benefit over dialysis. The prospect of renal transplant from HIV-infected donors into HIV-infected transplant candidates was first explored in 2007 in South Africa, where individuals living with HIV were considered poor dialysis and transplant candidates. Outcomes of HIV-to-HIV transplantation were found to be comparable to those in HIV-uninfected recipients, paving way for the development of the HIV Organ Policy Equity (HOPE) Act in the United States. Since the approval of the HOPE Act in 2013, multiple transplant centers throughout the country have been actively participating in a National Institutes of Health (NIH) trial assessing the safety and efficacy of this practice. While limited experience exists regarding HIV-negative to HIV-positive liver, kidney, heart, double lung, combined kidney-liver, and combined kidney-pancreatic transplantation, currently the research criteria developed by NIH for HOPE in Action only focuses on the HIV-positive liver and kidney transplantation due to ample experience with these organs.

Most transplant centers require the transplant candidates living with HIV to have an undetectable viral load with CD4+ T-cell count greater than 200 cells/mm^3 on a stable antiretroviral regimen (stable combination antiretroviral therapy [ART]). Additionally, transplant candidates should not have any evidence of active opportunistic infection and be on an appropriate prophylactic regimen following a history of opportunistic infections.

Pregnant or breastfeeding individuals are not considered transplant candidates; the same holds for patients with active malignancy, except those with Kaposi sarcoma, anogenital carcinoma in situ, or adequately treated squamous and basal cell carcinomas of the skin. Patients with a history of solid tumors (except central nervous system lymphomas) can be considered transplant candidates if they have received curative therapy and have been disease free for 5 years. All candidates with cirrhosis should be evaluated for evidence of decompensation and should only be considered for renal transplantation if eligible for a combined kidney and liver transplant. The patients with hepatitis co-infection should thus undergo thorough evaluation for evidence of chronic liver disease and advanced fibrosis.

With respect to donors, all donors must have no evidence of active opportunistic infections. Living donors with HIV must have undetectable HIV viral load and CD4 counts greater than 500 cells/mm^3 for at least 6 months prior to donation.

Following renal transplantation, induction therapy with lymphocyte depletion agents or interleukin 2 receptor antagonists should be commenced. Polyclonal depleting antibodies, especially antithymocyte globulin (rabbit) (rATG) have been used in renal transplantation. However, data establishing the safety and efficacy of rATG induction in transplant recipients living with HIV are conflicting. Studies have suggested increased risk of graft loss and infectious complications following rATG induction in transplant recipients living with HIV owing to profound decrease in CD4+ T cells compared to HIV-uninfected patients. The optimal maintenance immunosuppressive regimen is currently unknown, but generally includes a combination of (1) tacrolimus; (2) a mycophenolate analogue; and (3) long-term corticosteroids. Data support the use of tacrolimus as the optimal calcineurin inhibitor (CNI) due to its effectiveness in preventing rejection. Mycophenolate mofetil is a potent antiproliferative agent that confers the added advantage of HIV replication suppression. Sirolimus, an mammalian target of rapamycin (mTOR) inhibitor, has been shown to augment the activity of various cART regimens in studies in vitro and can reduce the progression of HIV-associated nephropathy by altering HIV gene expression in the kidney. Long-term corticosteroids are typically recommended to reduce the risk of graft rejection, the incidence of which is particularly high in transplants living with HIV.

Posttransplantation cART therapy confers a major challenge due to the risk of drug-drug interactions (DDIs) with various immunosuppressive agents for any solid-organ transplant. Patients with well-controlled HIV should be maintained on their pretransplant cART regimen after transplantation. Stable cART regimens should ideally include (1) integrase inhibitor backbone, such as dolutegravir, raltegravir, or bictegravir, given minimal risk of adverse effects and DDIs as well as overall superior therapeutic efficacy; and (2) 2 nucleoside reverse transcriptase inhibitors.

Tenofovir alafenamide is preferred over tenofovir disoproxil fumarate because of a favorable safety profile and reduced risk of proteinuria, hypophosphatemia, and renal dysfunction with concomitant use of CNIs. Significant DDIs exist with non-nucleoside reverse transcriptase inhibitors (e.g., efavirenz, etravirine, and nevirapine) and immunosuppressive agents, owing to their ability to induce CYP34A. Due to numerous DDIs and drug-related toxicities, such as hepatotoxicity, hyperglycemia, insulin resistance, and lipodystrophy, use of protease inhibitors (PIs) and pharmacokinetic boosters such as cobicistat should be avoided. Studies comparing the use of a PI-based regimen to non-PI-based regimens following renal transplants found increased risk of allograft loss and increased mortality in patients receiving PI-based cART. Hence, whenever possible, patients on PI-based regimens or those including cobicistat should be switched to an alternate cART regimen based on their resistance profile. In patients maintained on PIs or cobicistat, significant dose reduction of calcineurin and mTOR inhibitors is necessary to avoid drug-related toxicity. Use of maraviroc, a Cysteine-Cysteine Chemokine Receptor 5 (CCR5) receptor antagonist, in renal transplant recipients is currently being explored, and a theoretical benefit exists due to its ability to decrease the risk of rejection. It should be noted that resistance testing is strongly recommended before modifying cART regimens. Archival resistance testing in particular is helpful in determining a resistance profile in patients with suppressed viral load or low-level viremia.

Following renal or liver transplant, close monitoring of HIV viral load and CD4 counts is warranted. HIV RNA and CD4 counts should be checked 1-month posttransplant and then subsequently every 2 to 3 months to ensure virological suppression. Individuals with persistent viremia should undergo genotypic and phenotypic resistance testing.

One of the most common complications after HIV-positive renal and liver transplantation is increased risk of graft rejection, especially in patients with HCV-HIV co-infection. Studies have shown a 30% higher rate of allograft rejection in transplant recipients living with HIV compared to transplant recipients without HIV. The reason for this significantly heightened risk remains elusive but likely involves various mechanisms. Immune system dysregulation in transplant recipients living with HIV, inadequate exposure to immunosuppressive medications secondary to DDIs or dose adjustments as well as chronic immune activation associated with HIV have all been postulated as potential contributors to higher rates of allograft rejection.

Optimal timing of HCV treatment with direct-acting antivirals (DAAs) in liver transplant candidates who are living with HIV is a topic of much debate. While pretransplant HCV treatment can improve liver function, it can potentially decrease the likelihood of receiving a liver transplant. Given the particularly high risk of graft rejection found in HIV-HCV co-infected patients, current recommendations support treating all patients with lower MELD (Model for End-Stage Liver Disease) score and mild or moderate hepatic impairment with DAA before transplantation. For patients with MELD greater than 27 and/or significant renal impairment, treatment can be postponed until after transplant. Kidney transplant candidates living with HIV are eligible to receive liver and kidneys from HCV-positive individuals. The advantage of postponing HCV treatment until after transplantation provides the possibility of transplanting kidneys from HCV-positive donors, which is associated with shorter waiting time and expanded organ donor pool.

On the other hand, opportunistic infections and other AIDS-defining illnesses are relatively uncommon following HIV-positive transplantation. Instead, patients experience bacterial infections, with comparable rates as transplant recipients not infected with HIV. All transplant recipients living with HIV should receive appropriate chemoprophylaxis against *Pneumocystis jirovecii* pneumonia (PJP) as well as primary and secondary prophylaxis against other opportunistic infections according to national HIV guidelines (Table 22.1). The primary prophylaxis against *Toxoplasmosis gondii*, *Mycobacterial avium* complex (MAC), *Histoplasma capsulatum* infection, and cytomegalovirus (CMV) infection is based on the CD4+ T-cell count and follows the routine guidelines and recommendations as primary chemoprophylaxis in HIV. Lifelong secondary prophylaxis is recommended for transplant recipients with history of PJP pneumonia, *Histoplasma capsulatum* infection, and coccidioidomycosis.

All transplant candidates must be screened for latent tuberculosis infection (LTBI). Patients who test positive for LTBI in the absence of evidence of active tuberculosis should ideally complete treatment for LTBI prior to transplantation. Special considerations exist in transplant candidates with a negative screening test for TB but with a history of close contact with

TABLE 22.1 Management of Opportunistic Infections Posttransplant

Opportunistic Infection	Indications for Primary Prophylaxis	Duration of Primary Prophylaxis	Regimen
Pneumocystis jirovecii pneumonia (PJP)	All renal transplant recipients	Minimum of 1 year posttransplant Limited data exist regarding use of lifelong prophylaxis Consider discontinuation if CD4 > 200 cells/mm^3 for 3 months after 1-year posttransplant	*Preferred:* TMP-SMX 1 DS (800/160) or 1 SS orally (400/80) daily *Alternative:* TMP-SMX 1 DS orally 3 times a week OR dapsone 100 mg orally daily OR Aaovaquone 1500 mg orally daily OR inhaled pentamidine 300 mg in patients unable to tolerate other regimens
Toxoplasma gondii infection	Indicated in toxoplasmosis IgG+ recipients with CD4 < 100 cells/mm^3 Receipt of an organ from toxoplasmosis-seropositive donor	Minimum of 1 year posttransplant Consider discontinuation if CD4 > 200 cells/mm^3 for more than 3 months or longer	*Preferred:* TMP-SMX 1 DS orally daily *Alternative:* TMP-SMX 1 SS orally daily OR dapsone 100 mg orally daily + pyrimethamine 50 mg orally daily + leucovorin 25 mg orally daily OR atovaquone 1500 mg orally daily OR atovaquone 1500 mg orally daily + pyrimethamine 50 mg orally daily + leucovorin 25 mg orally daily

TABLE 22.1 **Continued**

Opportunistic Infection	Indications for Primary Prophylaxis	Duration of Primary Prophylaxis	Regimen
***Mycobacterium tuberculosis* infection (treatment of latent TB)**	Recipients with positive screening test for LTBI and no prior history of treatment for active or latent TB Close contact with person with infectious pulmonary TB in absence of evidence of active TB, regardless of screening result Donor with untreated latent TB	Treatment of LTBI should ideally be completed prior to transplantation	*Preferred:* INH 300 mg orally daily + pyridoxine 25–50 mg orally daily for 9 months OR INH 900 mg orally twice weekly + pyridoxine 25–50 mg orally daily for 9 months *Alternative:* Rifampin 600 mg orally daily OR rifabutin (dose adjusted based on cART regimen) for 4 months OR rifapentine (weight based; 900 mg maximum) + INH 15 mg/kg (900 mg maximum) + pyridoxine 50 mg weekly for 12 weeks in those receiving efavirenz or raltegravir-based cART
***Mycobacterium avium* complex (MAC)**	Recipients with CD4 < 50 cells/mm³ Active infection excluded	Consider discontinuation when CD4 count is > 100 cells/mm³ for 3 years	*Preferred:* Azithromycin 1200 mg orally daily once weekly *Alternative:* Clarithromycin 500 mg orally twice daily or azithromycin 600 mg orally twice weekly or rifabutin 300 mg orally daily

Continued

TABLE 22.1 **Continued**

Opportunistic Infection	Indications for Primary Prophylaxis	Duration of Primary Prophylaxis	Regimen
Cytomegalovirus (CMV)	Indicated if either donor or recipient is CMV IgG+ Prophylaxis is preferred over preemptive therapy in recipients living with HIV	Continued for a minimum of 3 months after transplantation Longer duration (up to 6 months) is recommended in CMV-seronegative recipients who receive organ from CMV-seropositive donors	*Preferred:* Valganciclovir 900 mg orally daily *Alternative:* IV ganciclovir 5 mg/kg daily
Histoplasma capsulatum infection	Indicated for CD4 < 150 cells/mm³ in recipients at high risk for occupational exposure or residing in endemic area	Consider discontinuation if CD4 count > 150 cells/mm³ for 6 months on cART	*Preferred:* Itraconazole 200 mg orally daily
Coccidioido-mycosis	Indicated in patients residing in endemic area with IgG+ or IgM+	Continued up to a minimum of 6–12 months after transplant; continued longer in patients with history of a more advanced disease; continue lifelong prophylaxis in recipients of organ from donor with history of coccidioidomycosis	*Preferred:* Fluconazole 400 mg orally daily *Alternative:* Voriconazole 200 mg orally twice daily after appropriate load OR posaconazole 300 mg orally daily after appropriate load

Abbreviations: DS, double strength; INH, isoniazid; IV, intravenous; LTBI, latent TB infection; SS, single strength; TMP-SMX, trimethoprim-sulfamethoxazole.

a person with infectious pulmonary TB and transplant recipients who receive organs from donors with untreated latent TB. Both of these patient populations should also receive treatment for LTBI. Significant drug interactions exist between the immunosuppressants and use of macrolide antibiotics and rifamycins used for MAC prophylaxis and treatment of LTBI, respectively, warranting close monitoring of immunosuppression levels. In patients maintained on a PI-based antiretroviral regimen, rifabutin dose should be adjusted to avoid toxicity.

KEY POINTS TO REMEMBER

- HIV-positive to HIV-positive solid organ transplantation is a life-saving measure with comparable survival outcomes to recipients without HIV.
- Inclusion criteria for recipients living with HIV include CD4 count above 200 cells/mm³, undetectable viral load on a stable ART regimen, and absence of any opportunistic infection or active malignancy.
- After transplantation, induction with interleukin 2 receptor antagonists or lymphocyte-depleting agents is preferred, followed by maintenance immunosuppressive therapy with tacrolimus, mycophenolate, and corticosteroids.
- Special considerations should be paid to the posttransplant ART regimens and DDIs with immunosuppressive agents. Preferred regimens include an integrase inhibitor backbone with nucleoside reverse transcriptase inhibitors due to a high genetic barrier to resistance and favorable side-effect profile.
- Posttransplant care involves close monitoring of HIV viral load and CD4 counts as well as screening for and timely treatment of opportunistic infections.

Further Reading

Blumberg EA, Rogers CC; on behalf of the American Society of Transplantation Infectious Diseases Community of Practice. Solid organ transplantation in the HIV-infected patient: guidelines from the American Society of Transplantation Infectious Diseases Community of Practice. *Clin Transplant*. 2019;33:e13499.

Harbell J, Terrault NA, Stock P. Solid organ transplants in HIV-infected patients. *Curr HIV/AIDS Rep*. 2013;10(3):217–225.

Locke JE, Gustafson S, Mehta S, et al. Survival benefit of kidney transplantation in HIV-infected patients. *Ann Surg*. 2017;265(3):604.

23 "I want to stop using drugs. What should I do next?"

Rick Elion

The patient JW is a 46-year-old African American man who had been diagnosed with hepatitis B virus (HBV) and hepatitis C virus (HCV) 12 years ago when he stopped injecting drugs. He was mixing heroin and cocaine after being unable to purchase pills. He had been diagnosed and treated for HBV with Truvada and for his HCV with ledipisvir/sofosbuvir. He was doing well but relapsed after being clean for 6 years. He enrolled in a treatment program with an opiate substitute, buprenorphine, as methadone made him tired. He found out he was had HIV when trading his dirty drug works.

He had stopped taking his medicine for HBV disease when he relapsed, and his physicians speculated that if he had continued on TDF/FTC (tenofovir disoproxil fumarate/efavirenz/emtricitabine), he would have remained HIV negative. His behavior resulted in acquisition of HIV, possible worsening of his HBV disease, and possible reexposure of his HCV disease.

What Do You Do Now?

CARE OF SUBSTANCE USERS WHO ARE LIVING WITH HIV

Recreational use of drugs and its impact on sexual practice and health is a phenomenon that has occurred over hundreds of years. The use of plants, synthetic chemicals, and medicines to alter one's consciousness and increase pleasure is an essential rite of life. I began to explore this topic 40 years ago in a defunct journal, *The Sensuous Hippie,* that explored the use of recreational and prescription drugs in combination with sex and found the most common drug (>70%) was nicotine, with alcohol and THC (tetrahydrocannabinol) close seconds and thirds, respectively. *Chemsex,* as it is now called, is one of the most common risk factors for HIV acquisition in our modern era and is a common route of disinhibition that results in less-than-optimal safe sex practices.

The use of drugs to change behavior is much more pervasive then even the common synergies of drug taking and sexual behavior. We live in an era of opiate addiction, a constant companion in the field of addiction that was fueled in the last decade by aggressive pharmaceutical marketing The impact of this addiction that drives drug-seeking behavior through numerous routes is destructive to the fabric of these individuals' lives and is dangerous to health through overdoses, supply and demand financing of oral medication, and the relatively tin ear of the medical establishment that has been slow to change prescribing practices or use opiate substitutes liberally. It is this backdrop of the normal human drive to get high, seek pleasure and run the risk of entrapment with addiction, and the incessant unyielding impact of desire that can cloud all logic that constitutes the background of this chapter.

The impact of addiction on challenges in holding employment, remembering to take your medications, and follow proper nutrition and a healthy lifestyle further complicate this picture. Add in the risk of obtaining drugs illegally with the concomitant exposure to the penal system, the drug treatment world, and the mental health complications helps create the context to understand the clinical challenges that patients and providers face when integrating all of these into the care of a person living with HIV.

People who inject drugs (PWID) have significant risks of acquiring HIV. Approximately 10% of all individuals living with HIV have intravenous drug use as their main risk factor globally.

CLINICAL MANAGEMENT

There is a certain hierarchy of questions related to the care of JW. The first relates to the timing of antiretroviral therapy (ART) treatment. The adherence to his medications will be critical to maintain adequate drug levels to suppress HIV replication. Does his substance use make it harder for him to maintain a schedule of taking his medications? This raises the question whether the goal for treatment of his addiction is to abstain from using drugs or to use his drugs in a way that does not jeopardize his general health or his HIV treatment. The philosophy of "harm reduction" is a well-respected notion in drug treatment and reflects the overall goal of stabilizing the health of an individual when the individual is not sufficiently motivated to discontinue drug use. This strategy seeks to maintain engagement in care and empowering individuals to abstain when they are ready, but to harmonize the priority of their health needs while continuing their drug use. This is demonstrated by using clean needles and exchanging needles rather than insisting that individuals discontinue their drug use. This is characterized by the use of buprenorphine or methadone, which is a type of substitution therapy, rather then discontinue heroin. Buprenorphine programs have been shown to be much more attractive to patients and so are considered preferable by many clinicians.

Adherence among PWID has been studied extensively and has been shown to be comparable to cohorts who do not use intravenous drugs. However, other studies have pointed out the difficulty in consistent engagement by PWID in clinical care. Only 31% were continuously retained in care over 8 years with less than a 6-month gap between visits. However, 85% of this same population did maintain HIV suppression less than 400 copies/mL.

A recent development in promoting harm reduction strategies is the concept of supervised shooting galleries. This first began in Vancouver, Canada, and the concept was to create a safe space for PWID to inject and provide them clean needles and a safe environment. The secondary goal was to eliminate the stigma of injection and create a judgment-free zone. This could eventually create a more supportive environment for PWID, and the people involved would be more open to drug cessation programs. Additional benefits were documented in many of these programs in different countries that resulted in reduction in drug use, retention in care programs, and potential decreases in mortality in patients who had been on methadone.

The patient JW has at least two diagnoses: HIV and his substance use disorder. It would be better if he had treatment for his opiate disorder to stabilize his behavior. However, small percentages of PWID are accessing treatment. Tsui et al. reported that less than 27.1% accessed methadone, and 5% of the population utilized buprenorphine in 2014 in the Seattle, Washington, metropolitan area, which has decent access to care and insurance. However, clearly access to insurance was a key factor in predicting access to opiate agonist therapy (OAT). Mlunde et al. performed a meta-analysis of studies that showed a clear correlation of OAT and higher rates of ART initiation.

Clearly, the goal is to stabilize the behavior of PWID to promote good adherence to their medications. However, it is recommended by most guidelines to start treatment as soon as the patient is able, which usually means as soon as possible.

JW had already been treated for his HCV infection, and his laboratory tests revealed a nondetectable HCV polymerase chain reaction (PCR) test. In patients who had previously been treated for HCV, it would not be possible to delineate an old infection from a recent infection with the HCV antibody test. Therefore, it is necessary to clarify if he has persistent HCV virus in his bloodstream, and the PCR test is the proper test to accomplish the identification of reinfection. The Department of Health and Human Services (DHHS) guidelines state that it would be best to stabilize his HIV infection and have his viral load less than 40 cps/m before initiating HCV treatment. The choice of the ideal regimen for him would focus on regimens that would be in a single tablet, as these have shown to be correlated with both higher adherence and higher rates of higher viral suppression. The current DHHS guidelines offer 4 different choices, and any of these would be acceptable.

The interval for the next visit and the counseling given at his first visit would emphasize making sure that either he is in an OAT and controlling his intravenous drug use or he is regulating his intravenous drug use to allow for consistent dosing of his ART.

The interval before the next visit should be short and could be 1 week or 4 weeks, depending on your comfort level that he will be adherent with his medication. The focus of the next visit would be to ensure that he is tolerating his new medications and that he is indeed taking them in a timely fashion. It is important to ask questions in a nonjudgmental fashion, such as, "How often are you taking your medications?" rather than "Are you taking your medicines every day?"

The choice of treatment for his HCV and HIV conditions is straightforward in most cases. As mentioned, the initial decision is choosing the optimal ART regimen. The most common choices include an integrase strand transfer inhibitor (INSTI) agent, which does not have drug-drug interactions, with the direct-acting antiviral (DAA) agents for HCV. So, any one of the DHHS recommended selections for first-line therapy will suffice. Use of the protease inhibitor (PI) class, which usually includes a booster, is not suggested due to interactions between the CYP3A inhibitor and the DAA agents, which could change the drug levels of the latter and result in worse clinical outcomes; therefore, it is best to use an INSTI agent with the DAA regimens for HCV. The clinical challenge here is not the selection of the specific regimen. The challenge is the engagement of the client with the provider and the healthcare system.

Parashar et al. reported in 2016 that the key drivers for morbidity and mortality were social determinants and barriers to adherence such as addiction, mental health, housing, and other similar factors. The integration of addiction treatment, harm reduction for those who do not wish to stop, and social support is the foundation of adequate treatment. There is not one formula that is right for an individual in the care of PWID any more than it would be for any other patient. The integration of OAT for those who wish to discontinue opiates, with the supplementation of harm reduction strategies for those who do not wish to discontinue, is key to providing judgment-free treatment.

A RETURN TO THE CASE

The patient JW has a viral load of 250,000 cps/mL, and his CD 4 count is 320. His genotype is wild type, he is positive for HBV antibody and HBV antigen, and his HCV PCR is negative. Despite his drug use, he was not exposed to HCV again, presumably related to his use of clean needles as he continued to inject opiates. Recent reports from Conference on

Retroviruses and Opportunistic Infections (CROI) 2020 by Clipman et al. showed the impact of networks contributing greatly to exposure to HIV and HCV. In their study, 42% of study participants shared syringes in the last 6 months, and 74% were directly connected to at least 1 viremic person in their network. This is a direct reflection of the risk of intravenous drug use that can be mitigated by either cessation of injecting or injecting with clean needles and syringes, reflecting the counseling provided to JW in previous visits. Factor et al. showed that sexual contact in a group of patients with HCV reinfections was the prime driver and not injection behavior. Finally, treatment selection of the ARV that was inclusive of an INSTI agent and nucleos(t)ide reverse transcriptase inhibitor agents, including FTC, was successful.

This case is intended to create the context, both socially and psychologically, of treating PWID with the medical challenge as the secondary goal. The cornerstone of therapy is to engage with the patient and as partners create a plan toward safer use of opiates or treatment of addiction with eventual recovery. Simultaneously, initiate therapy for his HIV infection for both the benefit of the patient and decreased risk of transmission to others. Six months after treatment, JW had been stable on a regimen of ARV and buprenorphine. He had missed very few visits and had not injected opiates since starting treatment. Let us keep our fingers crossed that this trend will continue for years.

KEY POINTS TO REMEMBER

- Care for PWID must take into account the medical needs (HIV, HBV, risk of relapse for HCV, possible need for opiate substitution) with the psychological and psychosocial goals of the patient.
- Adherence is critical for all regimens. JW had lapses in his TDF/FTC, which caused a resurgence of his HBV disease as well as a lack of HIV prevention that he could have been afforded from TDF/FTC, resulting in his newly diagnosed HIV infection.
- It is essential to identify the goals of the patient relative to the patient's addiction. Those who wish to continue using drugs

should be offered harm reduction strategies, and those who wish to discontinue should be offered a range of treatment pathways inclusive of opiate substitution therapies.

. The care of these challenging patients forces providers to be flexible and nonjudgmental in seeking to lead patients to a healthier path, with the understanding that their addiction will not be amenable to treatment until they are ready, and the provision of other medical services should not be impeded during this transition.

Further Reading

AASLD-IDSA. Recommendations for testing, managing, and treating hepatitis C. http://www.hcvguidelines.org/full-report-view. Version May 24, 2018.

Panel on Antiretroviral Guidelines for Adults and Adolescents. Guidelines for the use of antiretroviral agents in HIV-1-infected adults and adolescents. Department of Health and Human Services. July 10, 2019. http://aidsinfo.nih.gov/ContentFiles/AdultandAdolescentGL.pdf

Bell J, Belackova V, Lintzeris N. Supervised injectable opioid treatment for the management of opioid dependence. *Drugs*. 2018;78:1339–1352.

Clipman S, Mehta SH, Srikrishnan AK, et al. Explosive HIV and HCV Epidemics Driven by Network Viremia Among PWID. Abstract 147 presented at the 27th CROI; March 8–11, 2020; Boston, MA.

Factor S, Carollo JR, Rodriguez-Caprio G, et al. Sex, not drug use, is driving HCV reinfection among HIV-infected MSM in New York City. 27th Conference on Retroviruses and Opportunistic Infections, March 08–11, 2020, Boston; Abstract 594 presented at the 27th CROI; March 8–11, 2020; Boston, MA.

Malta M, Magnanini MMF, Strathdee SA, Bastos FI. Adherence to antiretroviral therapy among HIV-infected drug users: a meta-analysis. *AIDS Behav*. 2010;14:731–747.

Marshall BD, Milloy MJ, Wood E, et al. Reduction in overdose mortality after the opening of North America's first medically supervised safer injecting facility: a retrospective population-based study. *Lancet*. 2011;377:1429–1437.

Mills EJ, Nachega JB, Buchan B, et al. Adherence to antiretroviral therapy in sub-Saharan Africa and North America: a meta-analysis. *JAMA*. 2006;296:679–690.

Mlunde LB, Sunguya BF, Kilonzo Mbwambo JK, et al. Association of opioid agonist therapy with the initiation of antiretroviral therapy—a systematic review. *Int J Infect Dis*. 2016;4:27–33.

Tsui J, Birt R, Thiede H, Glick SN. Utilization of buprenorphine and methadone among opioid users who inject drugs. *Subst Abuse*. 2018;39(1):83–88.

Westergaard RP, Hess T, Astemborski J, et al. Longitudinal changes in engagement in care and viral suppression for HIV-infected injection drug users. *AIDS*. 2013;27:2559–2266.

Parashar S, Collins AB, Montaner JSG, Hogg RS, Milloy M-J. Reducing rates of preventable HIV/AIDS-associated mortality among people living with HIV who inject drugs. *Curr Opin HIV AIDS*. 2016;11(5):507–513.

24 "All of the above"

Anna B. Moukouri Kouoh, Nicholas P. Schweizer, and Glenn Treisman

ABCD is a 50-year-old referred to psychiatry for overall struggles managing his health. He has no reported family psychiatric history, with many admissions for substance use and suicide attempts. He exhibits odd behaviors, disorganized thoughts and poor eye contact and appears spacy. He endorses depression, paranoia, and active methamphetamine use. He is unsure of his psychiatric history and screened negative for contributory factors like trauma or brain injury. He has been to multiple treatment centers in the past 4–5 years, but relapses almost immediately on discharge. He reports periods of improved mood and diminished paranoia when off drugs and on psychotropic medications.

He was diagnosed with HIV in 1999 during a psychiatric admission. His follow-up has been inconsistent due to drug use, with poor antiretroviral therapy (ART) adherence; viral loads have ranged in the millions to currently 3200, and even down to 136 within the past year. He has been denied entry into multiple substance abuse facilities because of low CD4 counts.

What Do You Do Now?

MENTAL HEALTH DISORDERS

The diseases of addiction and mental illness are chronic health issues that are difficult to treat, meaning that patients often struggle for years to find effective treatment. The combination of one or both of these diseases with HIV can be devastating to an individual or even a vulnerable population. Mental health disorders have been known to increase the risk of acquiring and transmitting HIV, while having HIV increases a patient's risk of being diagnosed with a mental health disorder. In a literature review by Treisman and Pieper (2019), the prevalence of neuropsychiatric disorders in the population living with HIV is based on a variety of factors, which include direct effects of the HIV virus, preexisting psychiatric conditions, personality vulnerabilities, affective disorders, substance use and addictions, and other psychosocial issues, such as trauma.

Some of the most prevalent psychiatric disorders in the patient population living with HIV include mood disorders, schizophrenia, and substance use disorder. Psychosis is also discussed as this typically may present in the setting of all the listed conditions.

Mood Disorders

The term *mood disorder* encompasses a disruption in a person's emotional state leading to some disruption in their regular daily activities. Mood disorders can be grouped into three different categories: depressive disorder, bipolar disorder, and mania. Hindering effective treatment of person living with HIV (PLWH) with these comorbid neuropsychiatric disorders significantly increases the risk for HIV disease progression and mortality. Comorbid major depression is common with HIV disease, and HIV is well known to increase the risk of developing depression. The rate of depression in the patient population living with HIV has been estimated to be at least 2-fold that of the general population as HIV increases the risk of developing depression through direct damage to subcortical brain areas, chronic stress, worsening social isolation, and intense demoralization (Treisman & Pieper, 2019). It is reasonable to conclude that ABCD has a depressive disorder, as his reported symptoms of difficulty focusing, trouble concentrating, anhedonia, disturbed sleep, decreased energy, diminished self-attitude, and overall hopelessness are consistent with depression. In addition to these symptoms, he usually presents disheveled, with poor eye contact and speech that is typically low and mumbled; he can speak a bit more clearly if continually prompted to do so. At times, the patient even exhibits bizarre behavior, like checking in for appointments and leaving without explanation before being seen.

Bipolar disorder is broad in spectrum, ranging from a severely crippling and chronic mental illness to a mild disorder with alternating experiences of elevated or depressed mood, and the mania aspect of it is typically associated with impulsivity, impaired judgment, and risk taking, all of which can lead to behavior that accelerates HIV disease progression. ABCD exhibits impaired judgment and impulsivity, especially when looking at his drug use and poor adherence. Patients with mood disorders often present with symptoms that overlap with other chronic mental health conditions. In an article by Angelino and Treisman that discussed issues in comorbid severe mental illnesses in individuals living with HIV, they noted that there is difficulty in diagnosing bipolar disorder by history alone as the patients often present with depressive and manic symptoms related to their disease process or sometimes related to drug use; a reliable source may be required to make an accurate diagnosis.

ABCD presents with symptoms consistent with a depressive disorder and even possible bipolar disorder symptoms when looking at his bizarre behavior in the waiting room as reported, as well as risk taking that has led to his recurrent drug use and poor medication compliance. It is clear that despite the uncertainty of exactly what is going on with ABCD, there is a mood disorder component to his presentation and his symptoms, and when combined with his drug use, his compliance is worsened even more.

Schizophrenia

Schizophrenia in the patient population living with HIV is just as important as any other comorbid chronic mental illness due to the increased frequency of risk-taking behaviors in patients with schizophrenia alone. The prevalence rates of severe and chronic mental illness (historically encompassing schizophrenia and bipolar disorder) in PLWH are estimated to range from 4% to 19%, with no evidence suggesting that HIV causes schizophrenia, but data suggest that schizophrenia contributes to high-risk behavior associated with HIV infection. With schizophrenia, patients typically present with delusions, hallucinations, or disorganized thinking, all of which are positive symptoms. They can also present with negative symptoms consisting of emotional disturbances, which will affect the patient's ability to complete regular daily activities adequately.

In the case of ABCD, the clinical encounter may suggest there is an overall disposition consistent with schizoaffective disorder. The National Alliance for Mental Health (NAMI) website simply defines schizoaffective disorder as a form of schizophrenia that is characterized primarily by symptoms of schizophrenia, such as hallucinations or delusions, and symptoms of a mood disorder, such as depression or mania. In addition to the patient's reports of depression, he has on several occasions described seeing "shadows" moving around his apartment. He has periodically commented that in the evenings, things move around in shadows, but when asked to explain what he means and sees in detail, he withdraws and appears guarded. All of these symptoms are consistent with some aspects of schizophrenia, but even more aligned with the schizoaffective disorder variant, particularly when considering his mood symptoms.

Substance Use Disorder

In terms of substance use disorders and the population living with HIV, it is important to take into account the effects of substance use on high-risk behaviors, its effects on their physical and/or mental health, and its effects on the functionality of their ART regimen. The rates of substance use are significantly higher in PLWH when compared an HIV-seronegative patient population, with nearly 50% of PLWH reporting current or past histories of drug or alcohol disorders. The misuse of substances increases the chances of high-risk behaviors, such as sharing needles when using intravenous drugs, unprotected sexual encounters, not managing one's health (missing medical appointments, nonadherence to medications), and increasing the chances for abuse (sexual, physical, and/or psychological), all of which adversely affect a patient's treatment. Neuropsychiatric disorders are common in the population living with HIV and are based on a wide variety of factors, including direct effects of the virus, preexisting psychiatric conditions, personality vulnerabilities, affective disorders, addictions, or responses to the social isolation and disenfranchisement that can result from the diagnosis of HIV (Pieper & Treisman, 2019).

In ABCD's case, all of these increase the risk of him continuing to use, continued nonadherence to his treatment, and inadequate response to his psychiatric medications in particular. Drugs skew and distort one's perception, and the misuse of them can worsen symptoms, thereby making a diagnosis more difficult to treat and complicating one's HIV treatment. As previously discussed, this patient is at an even higher risk of continuing to or misusing substances due to having all of the risk factors mentioned.

Each of his health conditions increases his mortality risk, and the cumulative negative effects of them can be overwhelming, thus making it difficult for ABCD to manage even one of his diagnoses adequately. It is unclear how much of his symptoms, like paranoia, get in the way of his health management. His inability to make appointments on time and manage his medications limits his health outcomes; ultimately, it is difficult to manage him on an outpatient basis. In our clinical experience, extremely paranoid patients do not present with physical symptoms or may not report paranoid thoughts. They may present almost as shy and will hide what positive symptoms they are experiencing; this again makes it very difficult to treat the symptoms adequately. All these coupled with substance use compounds complexity in such cases and poses great difficulty with therapeutic interventions.

PSYCHOSIS

It is difficult to discuss the mental health conditions mentioned without talking about psychosis, especially in the context of PLWH and our patient ABCD. Psychosis is the loss of contact with reality, and it often presents as fixed false beliefs (delusions) and sensory experiences in the absence of sensory stimulation (hallucinations). These are all symptoms that may overlap symptoms of the mental health conditions previously discussed. Marder and Davis reported that psychotic symptoms can be associated with a wide variety of primary psychiatric and medical illnesses, making the previously discussed neuropsychiatric conditions of all mood disorders, schizophrenia, substance use, and others differential diagnoses for psychosis that need the underlying causes treated and ruled out. Depression and bipolar disorder can present with and without psychotic features; the hallmark of schizophrenia and schizoaffective disorder is the presence of psychotic symptoms, with mood symptoms for schizoaffective disorder, and substance use, among other things, often has to be ruled out in the setting of a patient presenting with psychosis as it could present with such symptoms. ABCD presents with both positive and negative symptoms of schizophrenia, a component of a mood disorder and substance use, namely paranoia, disorganized thinking, feelings of hopelessness, and poor eye contact.

CASE DISCUSSION

In ABCD's case, what makes it difficult to get a clear determination of his mental health diagnosis is that there is no clear evidence of a previous psychotic break, and there is no family history that can corroborate or contradict his symptom presentation. This poses the question of which of the patient's chronic illnesses came first. Is this a severely mentally ill patient who, because of his vulnerabilities from mental illness, was susceptible to and developed a substance use disorder, or was he a patient who likely had a mood disorder and the substance use worsened it? This brings us back to the initial question of whether the patient's presentation is consistent with major depressive disorder with psychotic features worsened in the setting of substance use, schizoaffective disorder, substance-induced mood disorder, or all of the above.

There is clear evidence of a mood component to his illness as well as co-occurring psychosis, and when coupled with his substance use, his symptoms are much more pronounced. Individuals with schizophrenia have been found to be more than twice as likely to have a substance use disorder compared with the general population, and with chronic use of substances, it may aggravate symptoms of schizophrenia, impede treatment, and result in more frequent acute psychotic episodes.

From the years of seeing the patient in clinic, we have determined that his symptoms coupled with his drug use are more consistent with schizoaffective disorder, depressive type, worsened by substance use. He has had multiple treatment modalities and has not shown sustained periods of complete symptom relief. However, he has shown better improvement when treated with a combination of an SSRI and an antipsychotic, especially with the usage of a depot form of an antipsychotic, also known as a long-acting injectable (LAI). A depot is a long-acting form of an antipsychotic medication typically administered via injection intramuscularly on a biweekly or monthly basis. This form of medication is available for typical (first generation, which are older, more sedative, and with more side effects) and atypical (second generation, which are newer, less sedative, and with fewer side effects) antipsychotics and is typically preferable in the setting where patients have difficulties with adherence.

ABCD is currently being treated with escitalopram, a selective serotonin reuptake inhibitor, and risperidone, an atypical antipsychotic available both orally and as an LAI. Patients are usually started on an oral dose of an antipsychotic medication and eventually switched to the long-acting formulation. This patient has remained on the oral and intramuscular formulations as he has continued to demonstrate extreme noncompliance with a medication regimen at each visit. He reported periods of improved mood and less paranoia and even presented with improved affect and appropriate behavior. His medication adherence and substance use were somewhat improved with better virologic response and CD4 count improvement, but this was temporary as he has continued to relapse.

Treatment of mental health issues combined with substance abuse treatment not only is key in mitigating or ending substance use/abuse, but also can assist with adherence to ART and address risk behavior disorders (Durvasula & Miller, 2014). Research has shown that patients like ABCD need simultaneous treatment of their chronic conditions. Patients with schizophrenia and a co-occurring substance use disorder should be stabilized with an antipsychotic medication at the outset of treatment; sequential treatment of the addiction first, followed later by treatment of schizophrenia is not recommended.

Despite his repeated relapse and continued low CD4 counts and detectable viral loads, the patient should continue to be treated in a multidisciplinary integrated care model. We have found it to be more beneficial to have more providers see him at 1 visit. Having the patient on a depot drug like Risperdal Consta that is given every 2 weeks allows for regular patient contact, so he remains comfortable, he gets more familiar with his treatment and providers, and in return, may help with better medication adherence.

· The diseases of addiction and mental illness are chronic health issues that are difficult to treat, meaning that patients often struggle for years to find effective treatment.

· Mental health disorders have been known to increase the risk of acquiring and transmitting HIV, while having HIV increases a patient's risk of being diagnosed with a mental health disorder.

· Some of the most prevalent psychiatric disorders in PLWH include mood disorders, schizophrenia, substance use disorder, and psychosis, and the patients often present with symptoms that overlap with those of other chronic conditions.

· These chronic illnesses need to be treated simultaneously when a patient demonstrates having all of them because they increase the risk of risk-taking behaviors like medication nonadherence, unprotected sex, and general mismanagement of health.

· It is very difficult to get a clear diagnostic picture of a patient with multiple chronic illnesses that are active and inadequately treated, especially in the midst of untreated substance use.

· Treating these patients in a multidisciplinary environment where all issues are addressed has been the most efficient and effective way to deliver quality care.

Further Reading

Andrew F, Glenn J. Treisman GJ. Issues in co-morbid severe mental illnesses in HIV infected individuals. Int Rev Psychiatry. 2008;20(1):95–101. doi:10.1080/09540260701861989

Campbell CE, Caroff NS, Mann CS. Co-occurring schizophrenia and substance use disorder: epidemiology, pathogenesis, clinical manifestations, course, assessment and diagnosis. 2019. UpToDate. 2019. https://www.uptodate.com/contents/co-occurring-schizophrenia-and-substance-use-disorder-epidemiology-pathogenesis-clinical-manifestations-course-assessment-and-diagnosis?search=schizoaffective%20disorder%20in%20HIV%20care&source=search_result&selectedTitle=8~150&usage_type=default&display_rank=8#H1238108609. Accessed January 15, 2020.

Durvasula R, Miller RT. Substance abuse treatment in persons with HIV/
AIDS: challenges in managing triple diagnosis. *Behav Med*. 2014;40:43–52.
doi:10.1080/08964289.2013.866540

Marder S, Davis M. Clinical manifestations, differential diagnosis, and initial
management of psychosis in adults. 2019. UpToDate. https://www.uptodate.com/
contents/clinical-manifestations-differential-diagnosis-and-initial-management-
of-psychosis-in-adults?search=psychosis&source=search_result&selectedTitle=1~
150&usage_type=default&display_rank=1. Accessed February 7, 2020.

National Alliance for Mental Health. Schizoaffective disorder. https://www.nami.org/
learn-more/mental-health-conditions/schizoaffective-disorder. Accessed January
7, 2020.

Pieper AA, Treisman JG. Depression, mania, and schizophrenia in HIV-infected
patients. UpToDate. 2019. https://www.uptodate.com/contents/depression-
mania-and-schizophrenia-in-hiv-infected-patients?search=neuropsychiatric%20
disorders%20in%20HIV%20care&source=search_result&selectedTitle=13~150&us
age_type=default&display_rank=13#H21. Accessed January 15, 2020.

Pieper AA, Treisman JG Overview of the neuropsychiatric aspects of HIV Infection
and AIDS. UpToDate. 2019. https://www.uptodate.com/contents/overview-of-the-
neuropsychiatric-aspects-of-hiv-infection-and-aids?search=neuropsychiatric%20
disorders%20in%20HIV%20care&source=search_result&selectedTitle=1~150&us
age_type=default&display_rank=1. Accessed January 15, 2020.

Pieper AA, Treisman JG. Substance abuse and addiction in HIV-infected
patients. UpToDate. 2019. https://www.uptodate.com/contents/
substance-abuse-and-addiction-in-hiv-infected-patients?search=hiv%20
AND%20addiction&source=search_result&selectedTitle=2~150&usage_
type=default&display_rank=2. Accessed January 15, 2020.

25 Silent No More

Rebekah Shephard and
Pamela Vergara-Rodriguez

Mr. Grue is a 58-year-old white male living alone in an apartment. After 5 years of struggling with depression, he is finally able to sit through a 90-minute Alcoholics Anonymous (AA) group without the dread of speaking with deep fatigue. At age 33, he received disability after an intensive care unit stay with HIV infection and PCP former abbreviation for *Pneumocystis carinii* pneumonia, now called *Pneumocystis jirovecii* pneumonia, PJP). He did not qualify for bankruptcy, so he went back to work and patchworked together several payment plans. His best insurance choice covers his medications, but copayments are tough. Now, he faces a new challenge: the cost of an alcohol-free meeting with a nice person. He saved for 2 weeks to cover the meal and transportation. Today, he can afford to go on his first "real" date. He comes to his appointment and nervously says, "I have a date." He is having second thoughts. He remembers the "I am an HIV-positive depressed alcoholic" announcement was always a roadblock to AA meetings. He states, "I am thinking I should cancel."

What Do You Do Now?

DEPRESSION

The prevalence of major depression among person living with HIV (PLWH) in the era after HAART (highly active antiretroviral therapy) is an elusive number. Before the antiretroviral therapy (ART) era, depression rates were as high as 80% and were largely associated with the neurocognitive changes associated with advanced HIV disease. Following the introduction of combination ART, rates vary widely due to the multiple subpopulations among PLWH: women, the elderly, men who have sex with men (MSM), youth, and injection drug users as they all face different mental health challenges. Depression has been associated with poor health outcomes for PLWH and the development of cardiovascular disease (CVD) and diabetes mellitus (DM). As seen in Figure 25.1, there is a complex relationship between biological and psychosocial factors and the development of depression among PLWH. Biologically, HIV viral replication in astrocytes, oligodendrocytes, and neuronal progenitor cells may play a direct role in predisposing one to depression. HIV viral replication creates a toxic environment of

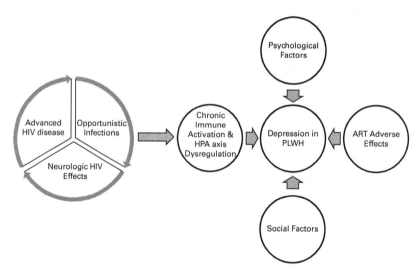

FIGURE 25.1 Factors contributing to Depression in PLWH

Adapted from Antidepresants for depression in adults with HIV infection (Review) Copyright @ 2018 The Cochrane Collaboration. Published by JohnWiley & Son, Ltd.

pro-inflammatory cytokines, a "chronic sickness" state that can be reversed with effective ART. Depression leads to biological changes that promote sickness effects on the hypothalamus-pituitary-adrenal axis and neurotransmitter expression as well as activation of pro-inflammatory cytokines.

Risk factors for the development of depression include female gender, being part of the lesbian, gay, bisexual, transgender (LGBT) population, older age, lack of social support, homelessness, food insecurity, and unemployment. Other psychosocial factors include isolation, discrimination, violence, hopelessness, and substance use. Certain personality traits, such as vulnerability, neuroticism, and insecure attachment have also been implicated. Psychological contributors to depression have largely focused on the burden of living with a life-threatening disease that is controlled but not cured, HIV stigma, and the stress of required daily adherence to ART.

SOCIOECONOMIC CONTRIBUTORS

What can we do about the concrete socioeconomic factors that impact a patient's overall psychological and emotional well-being? Many socioeconomic factors have been identified as risk factors for depression in PLWH, including lack of social support, homelessness, unemployment, poor income, and food insecurity. In a review of multiple interventions, reviewers found that relieving homelessness did not have a significant impact on adherence to ART, but depression was markedly improved. Food insecurity is positively associated with both depression and internalized HIV stigma. Unemployment and poor quality of employment may also contribute significantly to depression. PLWH who report adverse psychosocial work conditions reported similar depressive symptoms as those who were unemployed.

BIOLOGICAL CONTRIBUTORS: SUBSTANCE USE AND COMORBID MEDICAL PROBLEMS

Use of alcohol and illicit drugs is common among PLWH based on various cohort studies. Importantly, The *Diagnostic and Statistical Manual of Mental Disorders, Fifth Edition* (*DSM-5*) severe substance use disorder correlates with nonadherence to ART, more so than simply the use of a drug or alcohol. Depression has been associated with the daily, habitual use of alcohol; cannabis; stimulants (cocaine, crack cocaine, crystal methamphetamine); and opiates. Reduction of drug and/or alcohol use is consistently found to be beneficial for improving depressive symptoms and should be addressed whenever possible.

Comorbid medical problems. It is well established that patients with chronic medical illness experience depressive symptoms more frequently than the general population. CVD, DM, hypertension (HTN), and hyperlipidemia are all comorbid medical conditions that develop earlier in PLWH and partially account for an early aging process. In the CNS Antiretroviral Therapy Effects Research (CHARTER) study, depressive symptoms were found to be a predictor of distal neuropathic pain; both pain and depression demonstrated an impact on reduced quality of life. PLWH with depression also have more gastrointestinal (GI) symptoms (nausea, vomiting, bloating, diarrhea), which can limit the titration of selective serotonin reuptake inhibitors (SSRIs).

PSYCHOSOCIAL CONTRIBUTORS: ISOLATION AND LACK OF SOCIAL SUPPORT

How do isolation and lack of social support impact PLWH? The impact of isolation and lack of social support varies depending on the subpopulation of focus. African American MSM who have limited emotional support experience isolation and mistrust about personal relationships. They avoid emotional intimacy and instead seek physical intimacy through sexual encounters with multiple concurrent partners. The Women's Interagency HIV Study (WIHS) showed that social isolation and depression increased the negative impact of internalized HIV stigma, which led to decreased adherence to antiretrovirals. The impact of loneliness and fewer relationships increased rates of depression, alcohol use, and tobacco use in a study of older adults living with HIV. Overall, isolation and lack of social support have negative consequences for PLWH, so it is important to explore and encourage social connectedness for PLWH. Interventions for social isolation in PLWH include coping skills strategy, cultural activities, community involvement, knowledge education, peer group support, and support group interventions.

What is stigma? What can be done to reduce stigma? The Health Stigma Framework for PLWH identifies 3 HIV-related stigma mechanisms: enacted stigma (the experience of discrimination), anticipated stigma (expectation of stigma), and internalized stigma (acceptance of stigma as being true). Internalized stigma is associated with indicators of affective and behavioral health and well-being, while enacted and anticipated stigma are associated with indicators of physical health and well-being. Internalized HIV stigma has been negatively associated with poor ART adherence and increased mortality. HIV stigma is associated with avoidance coping skills and avoiding healthcare engagement. Interventions that target HIV stigma reduction and increased resiliency include strength-based cognitive therapy, cognitive behavioral group therapy, psychosocial support groups, and HIV-focused health education. Some stigma reduction interventions are population specific, such as LGBT focused groups. PLWH and depression may experience the stigma of having a mental health problem and related comorbidities, such as substance use disorders, social anxiety, and childhood and adult trauma.

SYNDEMICS

What is a syndemic, and why is it important? Being aware of syndemics allows you to prepare for your patient's unknowns. Syndemics are synergistic epidemics. In this case, we acknowledge that substance use disorders, trauma, and HIV have a high prevalence among MSM, transgender individuals, sex workers, youth, and minority women living with HIV populations (Figure 25.2). These syndemics and related behaviors (high-risk sex and/or behaviors, drug and alcohol use, and violence) must be addressed concurrently. Early childhood adverse events such as childhood sexual abuse, bullying, and family rejection influence coping skills and can manifest as depression, anxiety, isolation, or the opposite — being hypersexual and overly friendly or seeking attention.

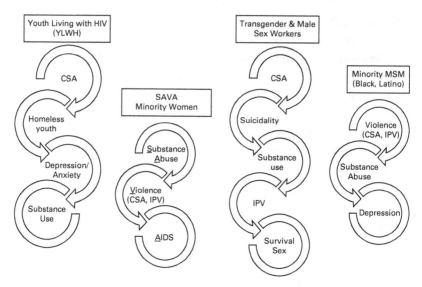

FIGURE 25.2 HIV Syndemics. MSM, Men who have Sex with Men; CSA, Childhood Sexual Abuse; IPV, Intimate Partner Violence.

For Mr. Grue, stigma is multidimensional as he is a MSM living with HIV with a history of alcohol use disorder and depression. Providers must teach patients that depression and addiction are chronic diseases. Providers need to promote recovery-based language such as substance use and depression "remission" and "recurrence" and avoid words such as "addict," "clean," or "dirty drop."

The U=U campaign is one potential answer to HIV stigma. The 2016 Prevention Access' Campaign U=U, Undetectable=Untransmittable, is an international movement among HIV patients, providers, researchers, and community activists to disseminate one important scientific message: *People living with HIV who are on treatment and have undetectable viral load cannot transmit the HIV virus.* This information has the potential to change the internalized stigma of HIV itself and it is hoped will allow a greater focus on other comorbidities, such as mental health and substance use disorders.

TREATMENT

Now that PLWH are living longer with HIV, quality of life (QOL) is more important than ever and therefore so is the treatment of depression. When we discuss the treatment of depression in PLWH, one cannot ignore the need for social services and psychological therapies that can target nonbiological contributors to depression in addition to the entire biological armamentarium.

Pharmacotherapy for Depression in PLWH

In a 2018 Cochrane review of 10 randomized clinical trials (RCTs) evaluating the efficacy of antidepressants, including SSRIs and tricyclic antidepressants (TCAs) compared to placebo among PLWH, antidepressants had a modest benefit in improving depressive symptoms; however, most of the studies reviewed were published prior to the year 2000. Importantly, medications were well tolerated, with the most common adverse effects of sexual dysfunction for SSRIs and anticholinergic effects for TCAs. In the Center for AIDS Research (CFAR) Network of Integrated Clinic Systems observational cohort, researchers found that approximately 40% met criteria (Patient Health Questionnaire-9 [PHQ-9] > 10) for the treatment of depression on cross-sectional analysis, of which 60% received treatment. The PHQ-9 (the patient health questionnaire for depression) is a 9-question screening tool utilized in both non-HIV and HIV primary care settings to identify both early and more severe symptoms of depression as well as suicidality. Duke and the University of North Carolina Infectious Disease Clinics were able to demonstrate validity and implementation of the PHQ-9 in their clinics for populations living with HIV, leading to an increase in the identification of depression. In the CFAR cohort, those who had persistent depressive symptoms after antidepressant initiation only a quarter received dose adjustments and even those receiving consistent evidence-based treatment, few patients remained in remission. This study emphasized the need for additional training and support to primary care providers to treat depression in the HIV primary care setting.

Choice of antidepressant treatment is largely based on safety and avoiding adverse side effects and drug interactions placing SSRIs as first-line treatment. In the current era of integrase inhibitors as first-line treatment for HIV, drug interactions are less important, and avoiding adverse effects is more important. Table 25.1 provides considerations in the choice of antidepressants.

TABLE 25.1 Considerations When Choosing an Antidepressant for PLII

SSRI/SNRI	Class affect: SIADH, gastrointestinal side effects
Drug Interactions with Norvir and Cobicistat	Paroxetine. Fluvoxamine, Vilazodone: CYP 3A substrates
Adverse side effects	Mirtazapine: weight gain, orthostasis sedation Paroxetine: SSRI withdrawal syndrome Citalopram: QT prolongation Fluoxetine: Long half-life (14 days) Bupropion: lowers seizure threshold and elevates blood pressure (BP) SNRIs and Psychostimulants: elevates BP
Comorbid anxiety/trauma and depression	SSRIs and SNRIs can be effective at higher doses
Comorbid substance use disorder	Antidepressants not effective in patients on Methadone with depression/ Combination of Sertraline with Gabapentin has found some benefit
Comorbid Insomnia	Mirtazapine: Lower dose is more effective Trazodone: may be beneficial as adjunct to an SSRI, as high dose of Trazodone often intolerable
Neuropathic Pain/ Fibromylagia Benefit	SNRIs, TCAs
Serotonergic syndrome	Tramadol, Trazodone
TCA risks and benefits	TCA Risks: Anticholinergic and cardiovascular effects. QT prolongation, sedation, weight gain TCA Benefits: Chronic and neuropathic pain
Cannabis	May worsen sleep health in PLWH May be associated with more GI symptoms

SSRI: Serotonin Selective Reuptake inhibitor
SNRI: Serotonin and Norepinephrine Reuptake Inhibitor

Testosterone: Premature testosterone decline hypogonadism is more common in men living with HIV, likely due to both medical comorbidities, including infections and disease, and as certain treatments. Treatment with testosterone is known to improve mood. Two meta-analyses of 27 RCTs demonstrated that testosterone replacement in those with hypogonadism can improve depressive symptoms (odds ratio [OR] 2.3) as well as QOL and energy.

Psychostimulants: Data on the use of psychostimulants for depression among PLWH is primarily targeted at fatigue in patients with HIV neurocognitive disorders. As such, psychostimulants may be most appropriate at low doses for patients with refractory depression or those with neurocognitive apathy. Comorbid methamphetamine and stimulant use disorders limit the safety of psychostimulant pharmacotherapy in the younger populations of PLWH.

Individual psychotherapy has an important role in the treatment of major depression. Among PLWH, interpersonal psychotherapy as well as cognitive behavioral psychotherapy can be effective in addressing beliefs and attitudes related to HIV stigma and self-efficacy. Videoconferencing may increase accessibility to individual therapy, especially among youth.

Psychosocial group interventions have been a mainstay of integrated whole-person treatment for PLWH since the beginning of the epidemic. The goal of HIV support groups is to provide a safe environment for disclosure and to process common experiences. A Cochrane database systematic review of 16 RCTs on psychosocial group interventions versus usual care in PLWH for depression found a small benefit for those with minimal symptoms but not for those with more severe symptoms. Three mindfulness-based stress reduction (MBSR) RCTs for PLWH have been conducted to address depression, fatigue, and QOL with overall benefit in terms of mood and affect. MBSR has been established as a benefit for several other chronic diseases, such as CVD, DM, and HTN. MBSR may be best suited to PLWH who develop other chronic diseases. Yoga has also demonstrated benefit for both depression and QOL in small trials.

Exercise: Studies in PLWH have consistently demonstrated the positive impact of exercise for both aerobic and resistance training. Best outcomes have been demonstrated with a combination of aerobic and resistance exercise 3 times per week for at least 5 weeks to improve several depressive symptoms and QOL as well as other physical parameters, such as adipose reduction and improved cardiovascular status.

Other Treatments: Patients may identify cannabis as a treatment for depression and anxiety; current studies in PLWH have not identified any benefits for depression or anxiety. Heavy or daily use of cannabis has been associated with more sleep problems, depression, and GI symptoms. Complementary and alternative medicine (CAM) therapies which include massage, acupuncture, homeopathy, herbal medicines, myofascial release and mindfulness, are common practice among PLWH. Though few interventions have been studied systematically, CAM therapies may improve self-efficacy and QOL but should be monitored for safety. Importantly, patients using herbal remedies should be cautioned regarding known potentials for drug interactions, specifically use of St. John's wort and SAMe (S-adenosyl-L-methionine.

Substance use disorder interventions for PLWHA include many of the same interventions for the general population, including cognitive behavioral interventions (used in intensive outpatient treatment); mutual help groups (AA, Narcotics Anonymous [NA]); residential interventions (28-day programs, recovery homes); medication assistance treatment (MAT; naltrexone, buprenorphine, methadone); and harm reduction interventions (needle exchange, Narcan for overdose). Most importantly, the advancement of ART has decreased the potential for drug interactions with MAT, namely, the integrase inhibitors have little impact on CYP enzymes. Several National Institute on Drug Abuse–sponsored clinical trials have been conducted in populations living with HIV, highlighting the importance of researching the best approaches to treatment in this group with multilevel barriers to care, such as housing homelessness, food insecurity, transportation issues, poverty, and poor social support.

The CHOICES (Comparing Treatments for HIV positive Opioid Users in an Integrated Care Effectiveness) Study focused on comparing intramuscular naltrexone to care as usual for opioid users, including no medication, methadone, or buprenorphine. Preliminary findings demonstrated that many social barriers prevent opioid users living with HIV from engaging in MAT or any treatment at all.

The HOPE Study (Hospitalization Visit as Opportunity for Prevention and Engagement for HIV-Infected Drug Users) utilized patient navigation with and without contingency management to improve HIV outcomes. This study demonstrated that patient navigation with and without contingency management was effective at improving engagement in care at 6-month postintervention, but lost effect at 12 months. This finding suggests that interventions are effective while they are ongoing.

KEY POINTS TO REMEMBER

- Multisystem resources are needed to address social isolation.
- Be prepared to address syndemics.
- Provide education about mental health, substance use disorders, and trauma.
- Change words and behaviors that can be experienced as stigmatizing.
- Practice trauma-informed care.
- Comprehensive mental health care involves medication and nonmedication strategies.

Further Reading

Eshun-Wilson I, Siegfried N, Akena D, Stein D, Obuku E, Joska J. Antidepressants for depression in adults with HIV infection. Cochrane Database Syst Rev. 2018;1(1):CD008525.

Nanni MG, Caruso R, Mitchell AJ, Meggiolaro E, Grass L. Depression in HIV infected patients: a review. Curr Psychiatry Rep. 2015;17(1):530.

Turan B, Budhwani H, Fazeli P, et al. How does stigma affect people living with HIV? The mediating roles of internalized and anticipated HIV stigma in the effects of perceived community stigma on health and psychosocial outcomes. AIDS Behav. 2017;21(1):283–291.

van der Heijden I, Abrahams N, Sinclair D. Psychosocial group interventions to improve psychological well-being in adults living with HIV. Cochrane Database Syst Rev. 2017;3(3):CD010806.

26 "Don't disrespect me, I'm Ms., not Mr."

Antonio E. Urbina

A 33-year-old transgender woman with male anatomy presents to your clinic interested in establishing HIV and primary care. She is originally from Jamaica was diagnosed in 2016. She received antiretroviral therapy (ART) in Jamaica, but treatment was inconsistent due to expense and trans-/homophobic discrimination by providers. As early as age 4, she remembers identifying as a girl. At age 18, she was tucking her penis. Her preferred pronouns are she/her. She is unsure of her previous ART but is currently on bictegravir/efavirenz/ emtricitabine (FTC)/tenofovir alafenamide (TAF) and reports that her last HIV RNA was undetectable and a CD4 of 520 3 months ago. She reports being on estradiol 2 mg twice daily along with 100 mg of spironolactone for the last 10 years. Because her current provider is uncomfortable with prescribing her feminizing hormones, she reports getting birth control pills from a girlfriend but would like to resume with her previous feminizing hormones and states she would like to transition her HIV and primary care to you.

What Do You Do Now?

TRANSGENDER WOMAN LIVING WITH HIV INTERESTED IN ESTABLISHING PRIMARY CARE

The management of transgender patients living with HIV is not too dissimilar to treating any person living with HIV (PLWH). Importantly, ART is recommended for all transgender people with HIV to improve their health and to reduce the risk of HIV transmission to their sexual partners. Infectious disease clinicians may be the first medical provider to evaluate a transgender PLWH. Available data report significant health disparities in this population, including increase rates of HIV, poor rates of engagement in preventive care, and challenges accessing necessary health services.

The prevalence of adults who identify as transgender in the United States is about 0.6%, or 1.4 million adults. A recent meta-analysis showed an overall HIV prevalence of 9.2% and 14.1% for transwomen and 3.2% for transmen. Another study comparing all adults of reproductive age found that transgender women have a 50-fold increased risk of HIV. Factors such as high unemployment, housing instability, discrimination, violence, and poverty all contribute to increased risk of HIV infection among transgender women.

As many transgender people have experienced stigma and past negative experiences, including violence, discrimination, and trauma, it is important that clinicians provide culturally and medically competent care. In fact, 40% of transindividuals attempt suicide compared with 8% of the general population. Before addressing any HIV-related issues, it is important that the clinician understand the top health concerns of transgender persons living with HIV. The most important of these concerns is establishing a connection with a clinician who is gender affirming and capable of providing nondiscriminatory care. Additional concerns center on access to hormone therapy, housing, mental health care, personal care such as nutrition, and last side effects of ART and their potential or perceived interactions with hormone therapy.

It is important that we provide transgender persons an opportunity to state their preferred pronouns as well as their preferred name. One simple way to start this process is to ask all patients, What is your current gender identity? We follow this by asking, What sex were you assigned at birth? Any discordance in these answers will identify a person as transgender. Next, we ask about gender expression, including preferred name and their preferred gender pronouns of she/her, he/him, or they/them if they should identify as nonbinary or gender fluid. Consistency in using preferred pronouns and name will help to build a good rapport with transgender patients. Last, we ask about sexual orientation by asking patients if they think of themselves as lesbian or gay, straight or heterosexual, bisexual, or something else. For example, a transgender woman who is sexually attracted to females will likely identify as a lesbian.

One of the top health concerns for transgender women is access to safe and affordable hormone therapy. For many transgender patients, gender-affirming hormone therapy is a greater priority than HIV treatment and care. In a cohort study of transgender women living with and without HIV, 64% reported use of feminizing hormones. Of those living with HIV, only 49% reported discussing ART and hormone drug-drug interactions (DDIs) with their provider, and 40% reported taking either ART or hormone therapy differently from prescribed due to DDI concerns. Data also support that transgender women were 3 times more likely to have an undetectable viral load and adherence to clinic visits if the primary care clinician was also a prescriber of hormone therapy. Because of this, transgender patients living with HIV should be made to feel confident that their hormone therapy will be continued.

HIV and ART are not contraindications to gender-affirming hormone therapy. Table 26.1 shows the potential pharmacokinetic DDIs between ART and gender-affirming hormone therapies. As shown, all nucleoside reverse transcriptase inhibitors (NRTIs), unboosted integrase strand transfer inhibitors (INSTIs), and select non-nucleoside reverse transcriptase inhibitors (NNRTIs) have the fewest DDIs and should be preferentially used as ART in transgender individuals. In the near future, long-acting injectable (LAIs) formulations of ART (e.g., cabotegravir and rilpivrine) will be available for both prevention and treatment of HIV. Importantly, it does not appear as if the LAI agents will have significant DDIs with either ART or hormone therapy. In this case vignette, the provider should continue the patient on bictegravir/FTC/TAF in addition to continuing with 2 mg twice daily of estradiol and 100 mg of spironolactone. For transgender patients on ART that interacts with hormone therapy, the provider should employ a harm reduction approach and continue with the patient's current hormone

TABLE 26.1 **Potential Interactions Between the Drugs Used in Gender-Affirming Hormone Therapy and Antiretroviral Drugs**

Potential Effect on GAHT Drugs	ARV Drugs	GAHT Drugs That May Be Affected by ARV Drugs	Clinical Recommendations for GAHT
ARV drugs with the least potential to impact GAHT drugs	All NRTIs Entry inhibitors • IBA • MVC • T-20 Unboosted INSTIs • BIC • DTG • RAL NRTIs • RPV • DOR	None	No dose adjustments necessary; titrate dose based on desired clinical effects and hormone concentrations
ARV drugs that may increase concentrations of some GAHT drugs	EVG/c All boosted P's	Dulasterde Finasteride Testosterone	Monitor patient for associated adverse effects; decrease the doses of GAHT drugs as needed to achieve the desired clinical effects and hormone concentrations
ARV drugs that may decrease concentrations of GAHT drugs	PI/r NNRTIs: • EFV • ETR • NVP	Estradiol	Increase the dose of estradiol as needed to achieve the desired clinical effects and hormone concentrations
	NNRTIs • EFV • ETR • NVP	Dulasteride Finastericle Testosterone	Increase the doses of GAHT drugs as needed to achieve the desired clinical effects and hormone concentrations

TABLE 26.1 **Continued**

Potential Effect on GAHT Drugs	ARV Drugs	GAHT Drugs That May Be Affected by ARV Drugs	Clinical Recommendations for GAHT
ARV drugs with an unclear effect on GAHT drugs	EVG/c PI/c	Estradiol	Potential exists for increased or decreased estradiol concentrations; adjust the dose of estradiol to achieve the desired clinical effects and hormone concentrations

The tables came from the HIV.org [DHHS] guidelines: https://clinicalinfo.hiv.gov/en/guidelines/adult-and-adolescent-arv/transgender-people-hiv

Note: See Tables 21a, 21b, 21c, 21d, and 21e for additional information regarding drug-drug interactions between ARV drugs and gender-affirming medications.

Abbreviations: ARV, antiretroviral; BIC, bictegravir; DIG, dolutegravir; DOR, doreminne; EFV, efavirenz; ETR, etravirine; EVGIc, elvitegravir/cobicistat; GAHT, gender-affirming hormone therapy; IBA, ibalizumab; INSTI, integrase strand transfer inhibitor; MVC, maraviroc; NNRTI, non-nucleoside reverse transcriptase inhibitor; NRTI, nucleoside reverse transcriptase inhibitor; NVP, nevirapine; PI, protease inhibitor; PI/C, protease inhibitor/cobicistat PI/r, protease inhibitor/ritonavir; RAL, raltegravir; RPV, rilpivirine; T-20, enfuvirtide.

therapy. Either changing ART or making dose adjustments to the hormone therapy can be made at a later date when more clinical and laboratory data become available.

Suggested baseline laboratory testing for this patient should include CD4 count and viral load; comprehensive metabolic panel; hemoglobin A_{1c} (HgA_{1C}); urinalysis; serologies for hepatitis A, B, and C; and screening for syphilis and genital, pharyngeal, and rectal screens for chlamydia and gonorrhea, if indicated. For patients on feminizing or masculinizing hormones, clinicians should also check a total testosterone level, estradiol level, and a fasting lipid panel.

Effective feminization in transwomen includes the use of estrogens plus a testosterone antagonist, such as spironolactone. Feminizing hormones result in breast growth, thinning/slowed growth of body and facial hair, redistribution of body fat and softening of the skin, and decrease in muscle mass. 17-Beta-estradiol tablets are the preferred formulation for hormone therapy. Ethinyl estradiol is a synthetic estrogen used in contraceptive preparations and is associated with an increased risk for venous thromboembolism (VTE). This patient should be counseled on the increased risk of VTE with birth control pills and restarted on 17-beta estradiol. Typical doses start at 1–2 mg/day with a maximum titration of the dose to 8 mg/day. At the same time, spironolactone at a dose of 50–100 mg should be started. Spironolactone is a potassium-sparing diuretic, which in higher doses also has direct antiandrogen receptor activity as well as a suppressive effect on testosterone synthesis. Hyperkalemia is the most serious side effect, but this side effect is rare when caution is used for patients with renal insufficiency or use of angiotensin-converting enzyme or angiotensin receptor blocker inhibitors. In such cases, switching to a 5–alpha-reductase inhibitor such as finasteride or dutasteride is possible.

Transgender persons may have elevated cardiovascular disease (CVD) risk due to both traditional risk factors and the risk factors associated with hormone use. Transgender women on estrogens may show an increase in serum levels of triglycerides and high-density lipoprotein (HDL), with a decrease in levels of low-density lipoproteins (LDLs). Transgender men on testosterone therapy may experience increases in levels of LDL and decreases in levels of HDL. Rates of tobacco use are higher among transgender people than in the general population, and studies have demonstrated that transgender women have a higher risk of VTE and ischemic stroke than cisgender men or women (people whose gender identity aligns with sex recorded at birth). However, many of these studies did not account for known health disparities among transgender women that can contribute to such events; for example, transgender women have higher rates of HIV and are less likely to be prescribed optimum medical management for CVD. In transgender women who have an elevated risk for CVD or who are current smokers or have already experienced a CVD event, transdermal estradiol may be the safest option for hormone therapy as it carries the lowest risk for VTE.

For transwomen, hormone level ranges should be in the normal physiologic range for a genetic female. When using feminizing regimens, the goal is to suppress the testosterone level to less than 50 ng/dL and reach a serum estradiol level in the physiologic, cisgender female range of 100 pg/mL to 200 pg/mL. When using masculinizing therapy, the testosterone levels should be kept in the usual cisgender male range of 400 ng/dL to 700 ng/dL. In this vignette, check testosterone and estradiol levels to confirm that they are in this range. If levels are out of range, then gradual up or down titrations of hormone therapy can be made over the ensuing months. There is no evidence that supraphysiologic estrogen levels result in faster or further feminization. In fact, higher doses may increase risk for VTE. Furthermore, some transwomen may request progesterone to assist with breast growth; however, this is not recommended as data have not shown this to be effective.

Another important concern for transgender persons is bone health. Bone metabolism is influenced by both testosterone and estrogen. Studies investigating bone mineral density changes in transgender women on estrogens have shown both elevations and declines in bone mineral density. The risk for osteoporosis increases after gonadectomy, especially if hormone therapy is stopped. Guidelines now recommend that transgender persons living with HIV be screened for osteoporosis using dual-energy x-ray absorptiometry by age 50. Also, since tenofovir disoproxil fumarate (TDF) has been associated with reductions in bone mineral density in persons living with HIV, non–TDF-based regimens should be used in transgender persons who are at increased risk for osteoporosis. Last, consider screening for osteoporosis earlier in patients not on hormone therapy, especially in patients who have undergone gender-affirming gonadectomy surgeries such as orchiectomy, vaginoplasty, or hysterectomy.

With this background in mind, it is important to perform an organ inventory during the clinical encounter with this patient as well. Transgender patients may use terms other than the anatomical names of body parts to refer to their bodies. For example, transgender men (people with male gender identity who were recorded as female at birth) may say "chest" instead of "breasts" and may use a variety of terms to describe their genitals. Regardless of the patient's gender identity, the clinician should wait for the transgender person to describe their body using terms that make the patient comfortable and repeat that language when referring to that body part. Transgender patients may also be reluctant to undergo a physical examination and may be wearing garments that help pad or compress their body into a more masculine or feminine shape. It may be important to only expose the body part being examined rather than to ask someone to change into a gown as this helps the patient feel as though they are less exposed and more comfortable during the examination. Last, when working with transgender individuals, clinicians need to remember that someone's gender identity does not determine what body parts (i.e., mammary tissue, a cervix, or prostate) they have or their sexual activity, and both should be ascertained in order to take a complete history.

Primary care for the transgender patient living with HIV does not significantly differ from primary care for the cisgender patient with the exception that gender identity and expression are not indicators of what body parts require screening. An organ inventory is an important part of history taking with transgender patients to assess what body parts are present and require appropriate screening. This inventory should specifically determine if the cervix, uterus, ovaries, mammary tissue, prostate, and testes are present as these organs all have significant implications in the care of the transgender patient or require routine screening that will need to be discussed with the patient. In the case presented, this transgender woman has male anatomy, including a penis, testes, and prostate, and all of those need to be considered when making clinical decisions regarding this patient's care.

Eliciting a sexual history from a transgender patient is important but can be difficult if either the clinician or the patient is uncomfortable talking about the transgender person's body. Mismatch in terminologies may result. As an example, patients may refer to the "front" of their genitals, meaning the penis or vagina, and the "back" of their genitals, meaning their rectum. Open-ended questions such as, What are the genders of your sexual partners? and How do you like to have sex? can help create an environment in which the patient can choose the language most comfortable to them to describe their bodies. These questions can help start a dialogue between patients and clinicians to open a discussion about specific sex acts and whether or not barriers are used. Answers to these questions can be used to determine the best practices for site-specific screening for sexually transmitted infections (STIs).

While hormone therapy does make conception more difficult, it is not a reliable form of contraception for transgender patients. Transgender persons require some form of contraception to avoid pregnancy during sex. Transgender women are encouraged to use barrier protection during insertive sex, both to prevent STIs and to avoid pregnancy if their partner is capable of becoming pregnant. Importantly, transgender persons living with HIV should strive for an undetectable viral load as a means of preventing sexual transmission of HIV to their sexual partners.

The most important times to discuss fertility preservation for transgender patients is prior to the initiation of hormone therapy and prior to gonadectomy. While hormone therapy is not effective birth control, it does reduce fertility, stopping or dramatically reducing sperm production in transgender women. Less is known about the effects of stopping feminizing hormone therapy in transgender women, though existing data suggest that sperm production returns to viable levels after discontinuation of hormone therapy. Transgender women should be offered sperm preservation options prior to initiation of feminizing hormones.

Surveys suggest that approximately half of medically treated transgender patients seek transgender-specific surgical procedures. Although hormone therapy is not a prerequisite for all gender-affirming surgeries, guidelines typically recommend the deferral of surgical procedures (other than transmasculine chest surgery) until transgender persons have completed at least 1 year of hormone treatment. Although the World Professional Association for Transgender Health standards of care and insurances require that a mental health evaluation be held prior to gender-affirming surgeries, the main role of the mental health provider in the presurgical setting is to determine psychiatric stability in order to ensure the best surgical outcomes.

Last, immunizations against infectious diseases are a particularly important component of care for transgender individuals living with HIV. When indicated, providers should ensure vaccination against influenza; hepatitis A and B; pneumococcus; meningococcus; varicella/zoster; measles, mumps, and rubella; and human papilloma virus (HPV). HPV vaccination for persons aged 27 through 45 years should also be considered in transgender patients, in particular transgender individuals who might be at risk for new HPV infections.

- Initiation or continuation of ART is recommended for all transgender people living with HIV to both improve their health and reduce the risk of HIV transmission to their sexual partners.
- As many transgender people have experienced stigma and past negative experiences with the medical system, it is important that we provide culturally competent care that includes the consistent and correct use of the transgender person's preferred name and pronouns.
- HIV and ART are not contraindications to hormone therapy, and data support that the continuation of hormone therapy by the primary care provider is associated with improved adherence to ART.
- Primary care for the transgender patient living with HIV does not differ significantly from primary care for the cisgender patient, with the exception that an organ inventory is an important part of history taking in order to assess what body parts are present and to assist with clinical decisions and age-appropriate cancer screenings.

Further Reading

AIDSInfo. Considerations for antiretroviral use in special patient populations. Transgender people living with HIV. US Department of Health and Human Services. https://aidsinfo.nih.gov/guidelines/html/1/adult-and-adolescent-arv/538/transgender-people-with-hiv

Endocrine treatment of gender-dysphoric/gender-incongruent persons: an Endocrine Society clinical practice guideline. *J Clin EndocrinolMetab.* 2017;102(11):3869–3903. https://doi.org/10.1210/jc.2017-01658

Radix A, Sevelius J, Deutsch MB. Transgender women, hormonal therapy and HIV treatment: a comprehensive review of the literature and recommendations for best practices. *J Int AIDS Soc.* 2016;19(3)(suppl 2):20810. https://www.ncbi.nlm.nih.gov/pubmed/27431475

Safer JD, Tangpricha V. Care of transgender persons. *N Engl J Med.* 2019;381(25):2451–2460. doi:10.1056/NEJMcp1903650

UCSF Transgender Care, Department of Family and Community Medicine, University of California San Francisco. *Guidelines for the Primary and Gender-Affirming Care of Transgender and Gender Nonbinary People.* 2nd ed. Deutsch MB, ed. June 2016. http://www.transhealth.ucsf.edu/trans?page=guidelines-home

World Professional Organization for Transgender Health. Standards of Care for the Health of Transsexual, Transgender, and Gender-Nonconforming People. 7th Version. https://www.wpath.org/publications/soc

27 "What shots do I need?"

Giorgos Hadjivassiliou and
Edgar T. Overton

In November, a 45-year-old man presents to HIV
care. He has not been engaged with healthcare
since childhood. He was diagnosed with HIV in a
local emergency room when he was evaluated for
atypical chest pain. He was found to have esophageal
candidiasis and given fluconazole treatment, which he
has now completed. His symptoms have resolved. His
sister was recently diagnosed with influenza. He has
not received a flu vaccination this year, and he asks
whether he should have influenza vaccination since it is
the flu season.

What Do You Do Now?

VACCINES FOR A NEW PATIENT WITH HIV

For persons living with HIV (PLWH), infectious complications are a leading cause of morbidity and mortality, attributable to the immunosuppression associated with HIV infection, particularly for persons with advanced HIV (i.e., when a person has a CD4 cell count below 200 cells/mm^3). The patient in this case has an AIDS diagnosis based on the presence of esophageal candidiasis, an AIDS-defining illness. This puts him at increased risk for numerous other infectious complications of his HIV disease. In addition to initiating antiretroviral therapy to prevent HIV replication and to facilitate immune reconstitution, there are key prevention measures that should be offered to him, including prophylaxis for opportunistic infection and certain vaccinations.

Vaccinations are a key prevention tool that can reduce the burden of infectious complications for the general population and have greater importance for immunocompromised populations, including HIV infection. However, the timing of vaccinations for PLWH is critical to optimize vaccine responses and to limit potential toxicity, particularly for live vaccines that carry the risk of reactivation, particularly in persons with advanced HIV infection.

Seasonal influenza vaccination should be offered to all adults regardless of HIV status and regardless of stage of HIV disease. The inactivated influenza vaccine is recommended for all PLWH regardless of CD4 cell count, while the live attenuated intranasal vaccine is not recommended due to concerns for reactivation in an immunocompromised host. While influenza vaccine responses are better in persons with CD4 counts greater than 200 cell/mm^3 and for suppressed HIV viral loads, influenza vaccination should not be withheld in flu season, as even persons with advanced HIV disease may receive a benefit from timely vaccination. As it takes 2 weeks for immune responses to develop, we want to give the influenza vaccine as soon as possible.

For other vaccines, administration can be withheld while the provider gains additional information about the individual's health status and previous vaccination records. In addition to the seasonal influenza vaccine, there are routine vaccinations that should be offered to all persons with HIV, including the conjugate pneumococcal vaccine, followed by the polysaccharide pneumococcal vaccine. PLWH are at 20-fold higher risk for invasive pneumococcal disease compared to the general population even in the setting of suppressive antiretroviral therapy. Due to high morbidity and mortality in this population group, current guidelines recommend the administration of the 2 currently available pneumococcal vaccines in series: the 13-valent pneumococcal conjugated vaccine (PCV13), followed 8 weeks or more later by the 23-valent pneumococcal polysaccharide vaccine (PPV23). A second dose of the PPV23 is recommended 5 years after the initial dose, and when the patient turns 65 an additional dose of the PPV23 should be administered. PPV23 doses should be administered at least 5 years apart. If the individual received a PPV23 vaccine prior to administration of PCV13, then the PCV13 vaccination should be delayed at least a year after the PPV23, with a booster dose of the PPV23 administered 5 years later. Other immunizations include booster doses of either tetanus-diphtheria or tetanus-diphtheria with the acellular pertussis component vaccination every 10 years throughout life. Also recommended is the quadrivalent meningococcal vaccination series based on the increased infection rates in PLWH, the high morbidity and mortality that accompanies invasive meningococcal disease, and the strong immunogenicity of the meningococcal vaccine. The meningococcal type B vaccine is recommended for certain individuals with increased risk of disease if they meet other criteria, for example, anatomical or functional asplenia, complement deficiency, eculizumab use, microbiologists routinely exposed to *Neisseria meningitidis*, and persons identified to be at increased risk because of a serogroup B meningococcal disease outbreak.

Regarding immunization against viral hepatitis, the 3- dose hepatitis B virus (HBV) vaccination series for persons who are nonimmune to HBV at a double dose (40 μg/mL) for each vaccine to increase long-term protection. A positive isolated anti-HBc (hepatitis B core antibody) in PLWH in the absence of positive HBsAg (hepatitis B surface antigen) or anti-HBs could represent either false-positive anti-HBc or chronic HBV infection with undetectable HBsAg or resolved infection. Those patients with a positive isolated anti-HBc should be tested for HBV DNA, and if undetectable, HBV vaccination series should be initiated due to the low anamnestic response in this population. Heplisav-B*, a novel adjuvanted HBV vaccine that requires only a 2-dose series, has not yet been studied in the setting of HIV but may replace traditional HBV vaccine in the future. In addition, PLWH should be vaccinated against hepatitis A virus (HAV) if nonimmune.

The human papilloma virus (HPV) vaccine series should be administered to PLWH under the age of 26. The safety of the HPV vaccine has been demonstrated in multiple cohorts, with evidence of seroconversion of at least 92% for each of the HPV strains among PLWH. HPV vaccine is an inactive vaccine and can be safely given at any CD4 count, but HIV plasma viral level of more than 10,000 copies/mL and CD4 counts of less than 200 cells/mm^3 have been associated with lower seroconversion rates. Despite the vaccination with HPV vaccine, patients should still be receiving age-appropriate cancer screening (anal and cervical Papanicolaou tests) because the vaccine does not cover all oncogenic HPV types. Finally, the vaccine is not contraindicated in those who have a positive DNA test, abnormal cervical or anal cytology, or genital warts since the HPV vaccine can still offer protection for HPV strains not encountered yet by the patient. Finally, the vaccine is currently not recommended for PLWH above the age of 26 years. One study demonstrated that the vaccine failed to prevent persistent anal HPV infection in men living with HIV.

If persons have not been adequately vaccinated against measles, this live-attenuated vaccine can be offered once an individual's CD4 cell count is confirmed to be greater than 200 cells/mm^3. This CD4 cell count threshold is relevant as the response for many vaccines is better for persons above this threshold. Fortunately, the majority of persons who were vaccinated prior to HIV infection (i.e., during childhood) retain immunity against measles, even for those individuals with CD4 cell counts less than 200 cells/mm^3. These data highlight the robust immunogenicity of these vaccines and the durability of the immune responses, even in the setting of HIV infection.

More than 95% of adults in the United States are immune to varicella zoster virus (VZV), mostly due to primary varicella infection (chickenpox), although a growing number of young adults received vaccination as children. PLWH who are unvaccinated are at increased risk for infection with varicella zoster at any CD4 cell count, but most notably when CD4 counts decline below 200 cells/mm^3. Additionally, elevated HIV viral loads have been associated with increased risk for incident infection and reactivation of latent herpes zoster infection that is abrogated with the initiation of antiretroviral therapy. Nevertheless, the risk of VZV reactivation is 3-fold higher in PLWH compared to the general population. There are very limited data demonstrating safety and immunogenicity of the recombinant zoster vaccine, but there are no data regarding efficacy in PLWH, and there is currently no official recommendation by the Advisory Committee on Immunization Practices (ACIP) to administer the vaccine in PLWH.

Some providers prefer to delay routine vaccinations until this threshold 200 cells/mm^3 and above is reached to optimize vaccine responses. The current ACIP recommendations only make this specific recommendation for live vaccines and for the polysaccharide pneumococcal vaccine.

Many providers develop a systematic approach to vaccine administration in clinic as part of preventive healthcare to ensure that all PLWH receive the appropriate vaccinations. Table 27.1 outlines some key baseline parameters that are relevant for vaccine consideration at time of entry into care.

TABLE 27.1 **Recommendations for Specific Testing for Patients at Entry Into HIV Clinic With Relevance to Vaccination**

	Rationale
CD4 cell count and plasma HIV viral load	These values have implications regarding timing of certain vaccinations that should be deferred due to immunosuppression.
Hepatitis A serology (HAV immunoglobulin G)	Demonstrate evidence or absence of HAV immunity and need for vaccination.
Hepatitis C serology (HCV antibody [Ab]) followed by plasm HCV viral load	Determine whether an individual has preexisting chronic hepatitis C, an indication for HAV vaccination.
Hepatitis B serologies (HBsAg, HBsAb, HBcAb total)	Determine whether an individual has preexisting chronic hepatitis B, an indication for HAV vaccination. Demonstrate evidence or absence of HBV immunity and need for vaccination.
Vaccination history	Ideally, providers should attain copies of patient's childhood vaccination records to determine whether they need specific vaccinations, such as measles-mumps-rubella or tetanus-diphtheria-acellular pertussis boosters.

- Seasonal inactivated influenza vaccination should be offered to all PLWH regardless of CD4 cell count.
- Other vaccinations should be administered within the context of the patient's HIV disease status and previous vaccine history.
- Vaccination records should be maintained for PLWH as part of comprehensive prevention services.

Further Reading

Crane HM, Dhanireddy S, Kim HN, et al. Optimal timing of routine vaccination in HIV-infected persons. *Curr HIV/AIDS Rep.* 2009;6(2):93–99.

Freedman M, Kroger A, Hunter P, Ault KA; Advisory Committee on Immunization Practices. Recommended adult immunization schedule, United States, 2020. *Ann Intern Med.* 2020;172(5):337–347. Epub ahead of print.

Kagina BM, Wiysonge CS, Lesosky M, Madhi SA, Hussey GD. Safety of licensed vaccines in HIV-infected persons: a systematic review protocol. Syst Rev. 2014;3:101.

28 "My gums are really red"

Fariba Younai

Sam, diagnosed with HIV 10 years ago, is virologically suppressed, with a CD4 of 451. About 1 month ago, he started developing nonpainful lesions in his mouth. He has a history of chronic anemia and skin folliculitis. Current medications are tenofovir disoproxil fumarate/ emtricitabine and raltegravir, duloxetine, tamsulosin, and Bactine spray as needed.

Clinical examination of his extraoral structures is remarkable for mild, nontender, bilateral enlargement of the parotid glands. He does not have any associated regional lymphadenopathy. Intraoral examination shows diffuse but well-circumscribed areas of leukoplakia mixed with significant erythematous zones. His oral tissues are very dry, and on gland manipulation, salivary flow from the parotid and submandibular salivary glands is minimal.

Incisional biopsies of the palatal and tongue mucosa showed a nonspecific mixed inflammatory response in the connective tissue and scattered fungal organisms on the epithelial surface. The final diagnosis for both biopsies was chronic candidiasis.

What Do You Do Now?

HIV, SEXUALLY TRANSMITTED DISEASES, AND ORAL HEALTH

Many sexually transmitted diseases (STDs) have manifestations in the oral cavity at some point during their course of infection and disease progression. For several types of STDs, the oral findings occur as the primary site of infection. Examples of these infections include (a) lesions of chancre in primary syphilis, (b) gonococcal stomatitis seen in gonorrhea, (c) the vesicular eruptions of herpes simplex virus (HSV), and (d) condyloma accuminatum of human papilloma virus (HPV). On the other hand, the oral cavity may be involved as a part of an STD spreading to mucosal sites. One great example of this is also syphilis, which in its secondary phase where lesions of mucous patch occur in the oral mucosa and in its tertiary disease lesions of gumma are seen in the oral cavity.

The clinical oral presentation of the STDs mentioned are similar to their presentations in the anogenital tissues and skin. For syphilis, oral lesions may be seen throughout the course of an individual's infection. After an average incubation period of 2 to 3 weeks, a painless papule appears at the site of inoculation of *Treponema pallidum*. Shortly after, the papule becomes eroded, and an ulcer of 1 to 2 cm in size with a raised, indurated margin ensues. This ulcer is the classic chancre of primary syphilis; it can last up to 8 weeks and is associated with regional lymphadenopathy. Figure 28.1 shows a chancre, a painless ulcer on the lower lip of 10-days duration. Secondary syphilis presents as diffuse hyperkeratotic lesions of mucous patch that may be found on the tissues of the tongue or palate, and gummas of tertiary syphilis present as painless granulomatous nodules found throughout the oral cavity and are associated with severe local destruction

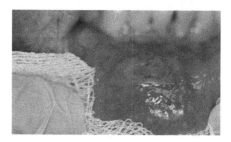

FIGURE 28.1 Chancre.

of normal anatomic structures. As seen in the patient vignette, diagnosis of syphilis can be challenging. Specific tests for immunoglobulin (Ig) M or IgG antibodies to *T. pallidum* should be administered if primary syphilis is suspected. Histopathology is usually nonspecific, and special stains such as Warthin-Starry may not be positive.

The pharynx is a common site of gonorrhea among men who have sex with men (MSM) and may serve as a reservoir for infection. In addition, nasopharyngeal infections may occur as a part of gonococcal dissemination. Pharyngeal infection with *Neisseria gonorrhoeae* is often asymptomatic, with no fever and lymphadenopathy, and sore throat is reported only with tonsillar involvement. Though rarer, primary infection of oral tissues, referred to as gonococcal stomatitis, may also occur as erythematous patches or ulcers covered by a pseudomembrane. It is interesting that oropharyngeal gonorrhea is self-limiting, with resolution of infection in the majority of cases, but because of its potential for spread to the genital tract and more invasive or disseminated disease, the condition should be properly diagnosed and managed. Currently, there are no nucleic acid amplification test (NAATs) cleared by the Food and Drug Administration for use with oropharyngeal specimens for the diagnosis of gonorrhea, but some laboratories have validated these specimen sites for clinical use. For the diagnosis of gonococcal stomatitis, histologic assessment of tissue samples from the oral lesion is used.

Oral HSV presents as a cluster of small vesicles that rupture and coalesce 2 to 3 days after their initial presentation. The great majority of oral herpes infections are type 1, but type 2 HSV is also capable of causing oral lesions. Figure 28.2 shows vesicular eruptions seen in intraoral herpes

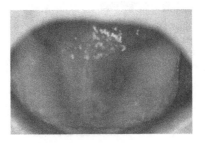

FIGURE 28.2 Intraoral herpes simplex.

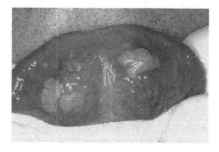

FIGURE 28.3 Squamous papillomas.

simplex infection. Recurrent HSV infection is usually manifested as herpes labialis on the vermilion border. Though uncommon, intraoral recurrences in healthy individuals consist of multiple, small, painless ulcerations that occur on the attached gingiva and hard palate. These ulcers also coalesce and heal within 10 days. In immunocompromised patients, recurrences may occur on nonkeratinized mucosa. Diagnosis of HSV-1 may be accomplished by histopathologic examination of tissue samples or by direct fluorescent assays and detection of HSV-1 and HSV-2 antigens in the superficial scrapings from the oral ulcers.

Oral HPV may manifest as squamous papillomas that are pedunculated papillary lesions (Figure 28.3), condyloma, a papillary lesion with a waxy surface and a very broad base (Figure 28.4) or focal epithelial hyperplasia that appears as clusters of a hyperkeratotic papules with a smooth surface (Figure 28.5). These presentations are benign manifestations of HPV-related infections. Though aside from the

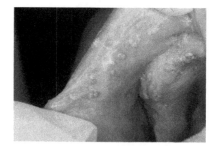

FIGURE 28.4 Condyloma accuminatum.

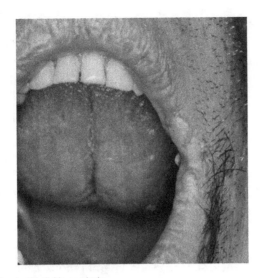

FIGURE 28.5 Focal epithelial hyperplasia.

systemic antibiotic treatments administered for syphilis and gonorrhea, no other specific treatments are necessary for their oral manifestations, as oral HSV systemic thymidine kinase–dependent antivirals such as acyclovir, valaciclovir, and famvir may shorten the duration of oral eruptions. On the other hand, HPV lesions are always treated locally by surgical excision, cryotherapy, or application of topical agents such as podophillotoxin and imiquimod.

HIV AND ORAL CANCER

People infected with HIV have a substantially higher risk of developing a number of cancers compared with uninfected people of the same age. Among these are 3 AIDS-defining cancers: Kaposi sarcoma, aggressive B-cell non-Hodgkin lymphoma, and cervical cancer among women. Although in the era of ART the prevalence of these cancers has dropped, people living with HIV are still at higher risk for other cancers, such as anal cancer, which people with HIV are 19 times more likely to develop, and oral cavity/ pharynx cancer, which is seen at a rate 2 times higher than in the general population. Oropharyngeal cancer is mostly squamous cell carcinomas (SCCs) with a variable clinical presentations that includes leukoplakia. Lesions are often painless unless they encroach on normal structures, such as muscles and neurovascular tissues.

Leukoplakia is a general term describing a white oral mucosal lesion that may develop as a result of any number of pathologic processes. Oral hairy leukoplakia (OHL) (Figure 28.6), hyperplastic candidiasis (Figure 28.7), and HPV-related oral lesions (Figures 28.3, 28.4, and 28.5) all appear as a leukoplakia and must be considered in the differential diagnosis of a suspicious white oral lesion. OHL is an Epstein-Barr–related lesion, first described in 1984 among patients with HIV infection and now known to present in many immune deficiency states. Pseudomembranous candidiasis is a superficial oral *Candida* infection that appears as white lesions and is usually easily diagnosed and treated unless a patient develops resistance to common antifungal agents. HPV lesions not only appear as white lesions that must be distinguished from dysplastic

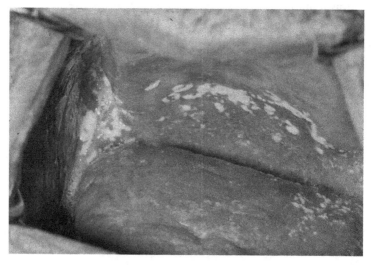

FIGURE 28.6   Oral hairy leukoplakia.

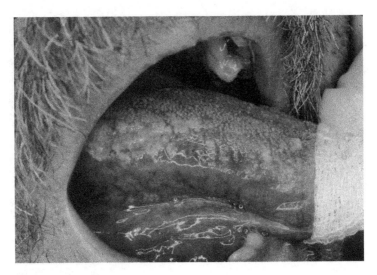

FIGURE 28.7 Oral candidiasis.

epithelial lesions, but also have a direct causal relationship with dysplasia development in anogenital and oral tissues. This is especially concerning among patients living with HIV, who have higher rates of oral HPV carriage. While an estimated 7% of the US population have oral HPV, this rate for patients living with HIV may be as high as 12.3%.

Other manifestations of oral cancer include nonhealing ulcers with indurated borders and exophytic lesions with high vascularity and nondistinct borders (Figure 28.8). The behavior of oral SCC is determined by the histologic classification, which consists of (1) well-differentiated, (2) moderately differentiated, and (3) poorly differentiated squamous cell carcinomas. When the level of maturation of the cells and their organization in the tumor tissue are close to normal cells, referred to as "well differentiated," the rate of growth and spread of the tumor is slower than when tumors are "poorly" or even "moderately differentiated." The diagnosis of oral cancer is always established by histologic assessment of tissue sample.

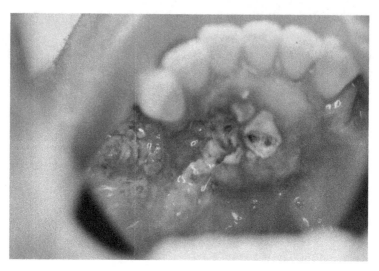

FIGURE 28.8 Oral SCC.

HIV AND SALIVARY GLAND DISEASE

Enlargement of major salivary glands and/or xerostomia (HIV-related sali-vary gland disease [HIV-SGD]) have been reported to occur in association with HIV infection. It is estimated that 5% of patients living with HIV de-velop bilateral salivary gland enlargement, and as many as 30% of patients develop xerostomia. Reduced salivary flow may occur as a result of HIV infection or as a side effect of medications used in the management of HIV disease and its comorbid conditions. HIV-SGD is believed to be associated with the BK polyomavirus (BKPyV).

Diagnosis of xerostomia is done based on the clinical examination of the salivary glands and their flow as well as the volume and character of whole saliva. Serologic testing for autoimmune markers is generally negative and rules out a diagnosis of Sjögren syndrome.

HIV AND PERIODONTAL DISEASE

HIV may be associated with specific periodontal manifestations as well as conventional adult gingivitis and periodontitis. HIV-specific manifesta-tion consist of (a) linear gingival erythema (LGE), (b) necrotizing gingivitis

(NUG), and (c) necrotizing periodontitis (NUP). LGE presents as pete-chial patches or as a uniform erythematous band on the free gingiva and extending into the attached gingiva; it is mostly attributed to infection with *Candida* species. NUG is characterized by rapid onset and acute pain, in-flammation, and rapid destruction of soft tissues, leading to necrosis of the interdental papillae. NUP leads to bleeding, sharp pain, and ulcerated and advanced loss of periodontal attachment, frequently leading to bone exposure. These findings are seen in association with very low CD4 count; therefore, with the widespread use of an antiretroviral (ARV) regimen, their presence in a patient living with HIV should be taken as evidence for lack of ARV use or poor treatment adherence. Figure 28.9 shows LGE as a result of poor adherence to the patient's ARV regimen. Today, the most prevalent periodontal finding among patients with HIV infection is conventional gingivitis and periodontitis.

Gingivitis is caused by the bacterial biofilm (dental plaque) that accumulates on teeth adjacent to the gingiva. Gingivitis is a reversible pro-cess and does not cause any damage in the underlying supporting structures of the teeth. Periodontitis results in loss of connective tissue and bone sup-port and can lead to mobility and tooth loss. Prevention and treatment

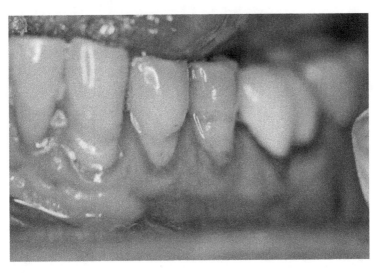

FIGURE 28.9 Linear gingival erythema (LGE).

of gingivitis and periodontitis focus on controlling the bacterial biofilm and other risk factors, such as smoking, and arresting progressive disease by antimicrobial treatment.

BACK TO THE CASE

Sam completes 2 rounds of systemic and topical antifungal treatment for *Candida albicans*; the treatment consists of fluconazole tablets and clotrimazole troches for 2 weeks, followed by itraconazole suspension for 2 additional weeks. After 1 month of antifungal treatment, lesions were not resolved. Two biopsies were obtained again and were examined for evidence of *T. pallidum* infection. The Warthin-Starry stain was negative, but Sam's rapid plasma reagin (RPR) test was high at a 1:128 dilution factor. Based on the RPR results, he received three intramuscular penicillin G injections within 2 weeks, and his oral lesions completely resolved (Figure 28.10). After the resolution of his oral lesion, Sam was started on cevameline HCl (Evoxac) on a daily basis for his xerostomia. His oral conditions and his medical status are both stable and under good control.

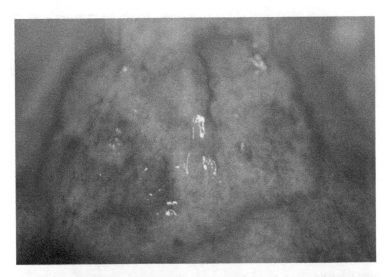

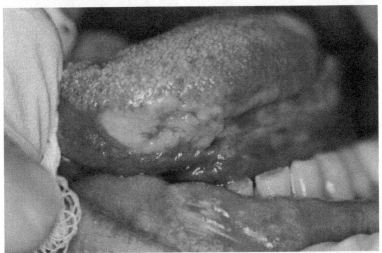

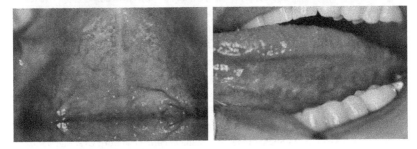

FIGURE 28.10 Resolved oral syphilis lesions.

Further Reading

Classification and diagnostic criteria for oral lesions in HIV infection. EC-Clearinghouse on Oral Problems Related to HIV Infection and WHO Collaborating Centre on Oral Manifestations of the Immunodeficiency Virus. *J Oral Pathol Med*. 1993;22(7):289–291.

Cohan DM, Popat S, Kaplan SE, et al. Oropharyngeal cancer: current understanding and management. *Curr Opin Otolaryngol Head Neck Surg*. 2009;17(2):88–94.

Cohen SG, Greenberg MS. Chronic oral herpes simplex virus infection in immunocompromised patients. *Oral Surg Oral Med Oral Pathol*. 1985;59:465–471.

Hernández-Ramírez RU, Shiels MS, Dubrow R, Engels EA. Cancer risk in HIV-infected people in the USA from 1996 to 2012: a population-based, registry-linkage study. *Lancet HIV*. 2017;4(11):e495–e504.

Little JW. Syphilis: an update. *Oral Surg Oral Med Oral Pathol Oral Radiol Endod*. 2005;100(1):3–9.

Jeffers L, Webster-Cyriaque JY. The probable association between HIVSGD pathogenesis and BK polyomavirus (BKPyV) has been validated with demonstration of HIVSGD-derived BKPyV oral tropism and proficient viral copying in salivary gland cells. *Adv Dent Res*. 2011;23(1):79–83.

Morris SR, Klausner JD, Buchbinder SP, et al. Prevalence and incidence of pharyngeal gonorrhea in a longitudinal sample of men who have sex with men: the EXPLORE study. *Clin Infect Dis*. 2006;43(10):1284–1289.

Murray PA. Periodontal diseases in patients infected by human immunodeficiency virus. *Periodontology*. 1994;2000(6):50–67.

Syrjänen S. Oral manifestations of human papillomavirus infections. *Eur J Oral Sci*. 2018; 126(suppl 1):49–66. Published online 2018 Sep 3.

Younai FS, Marcus M, Freed JR, et al. Self-reported oral dryness and HIV disease in a national sample of patients receiving medical care. Oral Surg Oral Med Oral Pathol Oral Radiol Endod. 2001;92(6);629–636.

29 Tray Tables Up, Ready for Departure

Gregory D. Huhn

WT, a 58-year-old cisgender man living with HIV for 25 years, with a CD4 of 553 and viral load of 250, and is enrolled in a long-term, nonprogressor study off antiretroviral therapy (ART). He is the director of an international gay travel company. Comorbidities include hyperlipidemia controlled on a low-dose statin; hypogonadism, currently addressed with testosterone replacement; recurrent herpes simplex virus (HSV) that has been treated 2 years by valacyclovir suppression; insomnia due to frequent travel; and latent tuberculosis infection (LTBI) that was detected on screening for dental work, for which he just completed a 4-month course of rifampin. His most recent viral hepatitis panel, collected just before initiating LTBI therapy, revealed a positive isolated hepatitis B core antibody, positive hepatitis A immunoglobulin (Ig) G antibody, and negative hepatitis C antibody. In 6 weeks, in February, he will lead a tour group mountain gorilla trekking on a 2-week trip in Uganda. He is requesting malaria prophylaxis and a 3-day fluoroquinolone prescription for self-treatment in case of diarrhea, and he asks if he needs yellow fever (YF) vaccination.

What Do You Do Now?

With global travel,[*] the intrepid can seize adventure, awaken discovery in the sublime, create meaningful relationships, build pride in accomplishment, and then tell cool stories. International tourism is growing; arrivals were 1.2 billion in 2015 and are projected to increase to almost 2 billion by 2030. Evolving trends in destinations through increased travel to Asia and the Middle East and with anticipated increases in travel to Africa will draw more attention to health-related factors with trips to these areas. Data from 2007 to 2011 from the GeoSentinel network of 53 clinics around the world point toward Asia (33%) and sub-Saharan Africa (27%) as the regions where most travel-related illness originate. Surveillance data and modeling suggest for every 100,000 travelers to a developing country during a 1-month stay, 50,000 (50%) will develop some health problem, 8000 (8%) will see a physician, 5000 (5%) will be confined to bed, 1100 (1.1%) will be incapacitated in their work, 300 (0.3%) will be admitted to a hospital, 50 (0.05%) will be air evacuated, and 1 (0.01%) will die.

Travelers visiting friends and relatives (VFRs) in their country of origin are at especially high risk for travel-related infections, particularly malaria and typhoid in Asia and Africa. Those VFRs comprise nearly 50% of US international air travelers, and they are less likely to seek pretravel health advice and view themselves with lower self-perceived risk; primary care providers may be unaware of their actual exposure risk.

In the United States, the foreign-born population is disproportionately affected by HIV. In 2010, while representing 13% of the population in the United States, foreign-born persons accounted for 16% of all diagnosed HIV cases, an important reminder to clinicians that person living with HIV (PLWH) VFRs should be regarded as having a similar, if not increased, risk of travel-associated infectious complications as US-born PLWH planning business- or tourism-related travel.

One of the first steps in deploying preventive measures for travel health in PLWH is assessing immunization needs based not only on risk of exposure, but also on the HIV-associated immune status (Table 29.1). As a guiding principle, for vaccination purposes PLWH with CD4 greater than 200 are considered to have limited immune deficits; however, seroprotection rates following routine immunizations may be lower compared to the general

[*] Assuming a degree of normalcy returns post-Covid-19 pandemic.

TABLE 29.1 **Vaccinations for Adults Living With HIV**

Vaccine	Type	Adult Dose	Route	Standard Schedule	Accelerated Schedule	Estimated Duration of Protection	Regions of Risk	Notes
Hepatitis A	Inactivated	1 mL	IM	Day 0 & month 6–12	1 dose prior for 40–60% immunoprotection when CD4 >300. Recommended immunoglobin for travelers >40 years arriving in ≤2 weeks.	24–40 y	Widespread	Higher rates of seroprotection with HIV virologically suppressed.
Hepatitis B	Inactivated	1 mL	IM	Day 0, month 1, & month 6–12	Standard dose HBV on days 0, 7, 21 for 38.7% seroprotection	>30 y	Widespread	
Combined Hepatitis A & B (Twinrix)	Inactivated	1 mL	IM	Day 0, month 1, & month 6–12	Four doses: days 0, 7, 21, and booster at month 12	>4 y	Widespread	
Typhoid	Inactivated	0.5 mL	IM	One dose	N/A	2 y		May have lower immune responses with PLWH
Polio	Inactivated	0.5 mL	IM	One dose	N/A	Lifelong	Afghanistan, Nigeria, Pakistan, Somalia, Democratic Republic of the Congo, & Papua New Guinea	Limited studies report 78–100% immune response rates among PLWH, with higher responses with CD4≥300
Yellow Fever	Live Attenuated	0.5 mL	SC	One dose, 10-year boosters for countries with entrance requirements	N/A	Lifelong		Should not be administered to PLWH with symptomatic HIV or CD4 counts<200
Meningococcal	Inactivated	0.5 mL	IM	Two doses: month 0 & month 2	N/A	5 y		Required for Saudi Arabia Hajj and Umrah
Measles, Mumps, & Rubella	Live Attenuated	0.5 mL	SC	One booster dose	N/A	Lifelong	Widespread; Europe, Venezuela, Brazil, Democratic Republic of the Congo, Indonesia, & the Philippines	Should not be administered to PLWH with CD4 counts <200
Japanese Encephalitis	Inactivated	0.5 mL	IM	Day 0 and between days 7–28. Optional 1-year booster	N/A	1–2 y, ≥6 y with booster		
Rabies	Inactivated	1 mL	IM	Day 0, day 7, & between days 21–28. Use boosters with expert advice if antibody titer low	N/A	Lifelong		Two doses required post-exposure: day 0 and day 3. Antibody response serology should be assessed with pre- and post-exposure prophylaxis
Cholera	Live Attenuated	1 Sachet		One dose	N/A	3–6 mo	Africa, Haiti, Yemen, & Southeast Asia	Should not be administered to PLWH with CD4 counts <200
Tick-borne Encephalitis	Inactivated	0.5 mL	IM	Months 0, 1, 2, & between months 9–12	Weeks 0 and 2, booster at 5–12 months, although immunity takes 3–4 weeks to develop	3 y		Vaccine not available in US or Canada.

IM = Intramuscular, SC = Subcutaneous

population. Seroconversion rates and geometric mean titers of antibody may be lower in PLWH than in healthy adult populations. ART partially reconstitutes the immune system by increasing B- and T-cell numbers and functionality, but deficiencies in humoral response may persist because of ongoing defects in memory cell function. International AIDS Society (IAS)-USA guidelines note that it is reasonable to readminister a vaccine or vaccine series 3 months or more after CD4 cell count increases with immune reconstitution on effective ART in a patient who may have a sub-optimal response to travel-related immunization at a CD4 level less than 200, including travel-related vaccines if there is ongoing risk exposure.

For PLWH, whether for tourism or business travel, some extra planning beyond immunization is in order, particularly regarding safeguarding antiretrovirals, to ease stress and ensure uninterrupted continuity of ART. Unfortunately, this travel checklist must also account for the 48 countries that still enforce entry restrictions for PLWH. Out of the 48 countries and territories that maintain these restrictions, at least 30 impose bans on entry or stay and residence based on HIV status and 19 deport nonnationals on the grounds of their HIV status. Some countries may require an HIV test or diagnosis as a requirement for a study, work, or entry visa. The majority of countries that retain travel restrictions are in the Middle East and North Africa, but many countries in Asia, the Pacific, and eastern Europe also maintain restrictions. In 2016, the United Nations Political Declaration on Ending AIDS called to remove all forms of HIV-related travel restrictions as these polices based on real or perceived HIV status are discriminatory, prevent people from accessing HIV services, and propagate stigma and discrimination. The following tips are helpful to secure personal access to ART, and for travel to countries with ongoing entry restrictions, these points can be modified as noted to prevent inadvertent disclosure.

- ART should be carried in hand luggage to preclude lost luggage, and extra days of medications are encouraged in case return plans are disrupted.
- Though in virtually all cases importing medicines for personal use should not pose a problem, a traveler should carry a doctor's prescription in English, importantly with no mention of HIV.
- ART should be in original packaging, labeled with the traveler's name.
  - In a country with restrictions, ART should be rebottled in neutral packaging without the name of the medication. To comply with laws in many countries, the same letter from the provider without mentioning HIV should state these medications are for a personal medical condition.

- HIV status should not be disclosed unnecessarily to customs or immigration officials, or other unfamiliar travelers, to avoid stigmatization in some countries.
- If staying in a country for a longer period, or if a medical problem arises, knowledge of a nearby HIV clinic is useful, as is establishing communication with a local HIV organization.
  - The last dose of ART should be taken before checking in as possession of medications in hand luggage in a country with restrictions is not without risk of country-specific penalties.

Importantly, PLWH need to be aware that perceptions around HIV infection change from country to country. If disclosure is safe in the country or community called home, this may not be the case in the foreign travel destination.

Pretravel consultation should take place at least 6 to 8 weeks before departure, and PLWH may require additional nontravel vaccines compared to the general population. All travelers are at risk for respiratory illnesses from person-to-person transmission, so seasonal influenza and pneumococcal immunization should be initiated or updated if not already administered. A compendium of travel health preventive issues among PLWH is presented to provide general information specific to the most common considerations for malaria prophylaxis, vaccination, and traveler's diarrhea.

MALARIA

Travelers to malarial zones should first grasp methods for preventing bites from *Anopheles* mosquitoes. Guidance includes avoiding outdoor exposure between dusk and dawn when *Anopheles* mosquitoes feed for a blood meal, wearing clothing that covers exposed skin, using insect repellant, sleeping within permethrin bed nets, and trying to stay in well-screened or air-conditioned rooms, particularly during nocturnal hours. For insect repellents the Centers for Disease Control and Prevention (CDC) recommends *N,N*-diethyl-m-toluamide (DEET), picaridin, ethyl butylacetylaminopropionate (IR3535), or oil of lemon eucalyptus. Clothing and bed netting treated with permethrin effectively repel mosquitoes for more than a week, even with washing and field use.

For chemoprophylaxis, the most recent CDC and World Health Organization (WHO) guidelines and advisories for malaria transmission regions should be reviewed together with itineraries to determine the appropriate approach to chemoprophylaxis. For destinations with only sporadic malaria activity and risk to travelers is regarded as very low, mosquito avoidance measures can be used alone as chemoprophylaxis is generally not needed. For travelers at risk of exposure in areas where chloroquine-resistant *Plasmodium falciparum* malaria is present, mosquito avoidance should be used in conjunction with chemoprophylaxis. There are 4 agents that are highly efficacious for malaria prevention, specifically atovaquone-proguanil, mefloquine, doxycycline, and tafenoquine, and each has unique characteristics, including potential drug-drug interactions with antiretrovirals, that should be considered in PLWH (Table 29.2). Additionally, for PLWH some experts recommend trimethoprim-sulfamethoxazole (SMX-TMP) for prevention of malaria regardless of CD4 count if living long term in malaria-endemic areas, with studies from Uganda demonstrating reduced morbidity and mortality rates due to malaria in PLWH taking SMX-TMP prophylaxis, even in areas with a high rate of malaria resistance.

TABLE 29.2 **Malaria Prophylaxis Adults Living With HIV**

Region of Risk	Medication	Adult Dose	Standard Schedule	Drug x Drug Interactions	Notes
	Atovaquone-proguanil	250 mg atovaquone & 100 mg proguanil	1 dose daily, initiate 1–2 days prior to arrival, continue daily throughout stay and 7 days after	Concomitant dapsone may increase risk for hemolytic reactions. Efavirenz may decrease serum concentration of atovaquone, consider alternative antimalarial prophylaxis. Ritonavir may decrease serum concentration of atovoquone and proguanil.	May be preferred for short term travel. Not indicated with CrCl < 30 mL/minute
	Mefloquine	250 mg	1 dose weekly, initiate 1 week prior to arrival, continue weekly throughout and 4 weeks after	Concomitant dapsone may increase the risk of hemolytic reactions. Concentrations may be affected by CYP3A4 inducer and inhibitor antiretroviral medications.	May be preferred for long term travel
	Doxycycline	100 mg	1 dose daily 1 to 2 days prior to arrival, continue daily throughout stay and 4 weeks after	N/A	Associated with sun sensitization, may increase risk of rash, itchiness, sunburn
	Tafenoquine	200 mg	Loading 200 mg dose daily 3 days prior to arrival, continue 200 mg weekly dose throughout, starting 7 days after arrival. Single 200 mg dose 7 days after return.	N/A	May be preferred for short term or last-minute travel. Can cause severe hemolytic anemia in PLWH with G6PD deficiency; use quantitative G6PD test to rule out deficiency prior to administration of drug

G6PD, glucose-6-phosphate dehydrogenase.

YELLOW FEVER

Perhaps no other preventive health measure in international travel generates more debate than YF vaccination, especially for PLWH. YF is an arboviral flavivirus infection transmitted by *Aedes* mosquitoes in the "yellow fever belt" endemic zone in sub-Saharan Africa and South America, latitudes approximately 15° north and 10° south, with recent urban outbreaks creeping into major metropolitan cities along the Brazilian coastline. The risk of overall YF transmission is estimated to be low (between < 1 per 1,000,000 and < 1,100,000), but for those who acquire YF and develop hemorrhagic fever complications, it is a lethal disease, with up to a 90% case-fatality rate. In addition to its indication for preventing infection in individuals at risk, be it populations living in an endemic area or travelers, it is the only vaccine currently under the WHO's International Health Regulations (IHR) that may necessitate vaccination for its other overarching goal, to prevent international spread by minimizing the risk of importation of the virus by asymptomatic viremic travelers.

Whether PLWH have a higher risk of acquisition or more severe YF illness is unknown. The live attenuated vaccine itself is highly effective, but because of rare but serious vaccine-associated events (1 per 334,000 doses), namely viscerotropic or neurotropic reactions that mimic wild-type virus disease from reversion of the live attenuated vaccine, which occur most frequently in persons aged 60 years or older or persons with thymic disorders, individuals not at any risk of exposure should not be vaccinated. Decisions about YF vaccination are conditioned on risk-benefit assessment for the traveler, the itinerary, and destination country entry requirements. Several African countries and French Guiana in South America require proof of YF vaccination from all arriving travelers, and other countries, both within and outside risk zones, have more complex requirements for airplane connection or other transportation transit of travelers arriving directly or via a country in a YF endemic zone, but not from travelers arriving from countries outside these zones. Current country-by-country YF entry requirements are available from the WHO.

Yellow fever vaccination is only available from designated centers in the United States authorized by state health departments to legally stamp an international certification of vaccination. For PLWH, WHO guidelines state that YF vaccine may be offered to asymptomatic persons with CD4 200 or greater, and in cases of symptomatic HIV or those with CD4 counts less than 200, the vaccine should not be administered. US guidelines recommend that PLWH should ideally avoid traveling to YF endemic zones, but the vaccine can be offered if travel itineraries put the person anywhere close to regions with risk of YF arboviral transmission.

Specifically, YF vaccination is a precaution for asymptomatic HIV-infected persons with CD4 cell counts of 200–499; hence, the benefits and risks should be carefully discussed. And, vaccination is not a precaution for PLWH with CD4 cell counts 500 or greater. Vaccine recipients should be monitored closely for possible adverse effects; however, no cases of postvaccination viscerotropic disease in PLWH have been reported to date, and PLWH with virologic suppression respond well to YF immunization regardless of CD4 count. Because vaccine response may nonetheless by suboptimal, serological testing for immune response may be checked 1 month following vaccination.

If the only reason to vaccinate is for international travel requirements, and not actual exposure risk, then any PLWH should request a written "waiver letter" from their clinician stating the reasons for exemption. A word of caution, though, with this strategy, the destination country may quarantine the traveler on arrival for up to 6 days or place the traveler under surveillance during their stay. Variations in exposure risk within endemic regions (an area of risk may be restricted to only a portion of the country) must be considered, and travel should be canceled if the risk of exposure is more than negligible and YF vaccine cannot be administered or is declined for the PLWH.

Regarding immune responses to YF vaccination, PLWH have lower vaccine response rates compared to HIV-uninfected persons based on studies, including a Cochrane review. One study showed that 83% developed neutralizing antibody compared with 97% of HIV-uninfected persons ($p = .01$), with immune responses greater among those with higher CD4 counts and lower HIV viral loads. Another study found that 98% of PLWH had an initial seroresponse, which decreased to 92% at 10 years postvaccination, with durability being closely related to suppressed HIV viral loads over time.

The conventional understanding that YF vaccination provided protection for 10 years has now been superseded by more recent CDC analyses that 80% of healthy vaccines have virus-neutralizing antibodies 20 years postvaccination, connoting long-term immunity, and for IHR purposes documentation of a single YF vaccine at any time during a person's life should suffice for entry for any country requirements. That being said, the CDC recommends that 10-year booster vaccination should be extended to healthy travelers planning a long stay in any county with risk of transmission; all travelers spending any amount of time in high-risk areas, notably West Africa; and all persons traveling to an area with an ongoing outbreak. For PLWH who continue to be at risk over a long period of time, guidelines suggest revaccination every 10 years. Finally, a YF certificate becomes valid for country entry 10 days after it was stamped and dated, the approximate time frame for establishing seroprotection postvaccination.

HEPATITIS A

Hepatitis A vaccination is recommended for all nonimmune PLWH as routine vaccination. Hepatitis A infection is one of the most common vaccine-preventable diseases encountered by travelers. Of all reported hepatitis A infections in 2006 with identifiable risk factors in the United States, 14.7% (196/1337) were attributed to exposure during international travel. Trip characteristics suggesting particularly high risk include destinations with poor hygiene and sanitation practices and adventurous eating habits. For last-minute travel, 1 dose without the booster can generate immunoprotection in 40%–60% of PLWH when the CD4 is greater than 200–300. The CDC recommends ancillary concomitant immunoglobulin for travelers older 40 years of age, including PLWH, who are planning to depart in 2 weeks or less, though this practice has not been widely adopted. For time-constrained travelers, there are limited data to suggest that alternative dosing strategies (e.g., administering a second dose of hepatitis A vaccine at least 4 weeks after the first dose or a combined hepatitis A and hepatitis B [Twinrix] 3-dose rapid schedule at 0, 1, and 3 weeks) are effective strategies. For this combined vaccine, however, there are no data for seroprotection rates among PLWH using the accelerated dosing schedule. For PLWH, there was a 7-fold higher rate of seroprotection if HIV was virologically suppressed, and response rates were greater if the 3-dose series was completed versus incomplete (62% vs. 40%). Efforts should be made to compete booster doses for hepatitis A immunization once travel is complete.

HEPATITIS B

Hepatitis B vaccination is recommended for all nonimmune PLWH as routine vaccination. Risk factors for blood-borne or sexual exposure include adventure travel; medical tourism; or health condition that may warrant medical intervention, injections, or infusions. Approximately 10%–15% of international travelers in surveys reported contact with blood or other body fluids. For last-minute travel, an accelerated 3-week schedule with conventional standard dose hepatitis at 0, 7, and 21 days may be considered, although seroprotection in PLWH is only 38.7%. There are no hepatitis B seroprotection data in PLWH with the combined hepatitis A and hepatitis B (Twinrix) accelerated dose schedule. Tenofovir with lamivudine or emtricitabine in several ART regimens is recognized as prophylaxis against hepatitis B.

TYPHOID

There are 2 vaccines against *Salmonella enterica* serovar Typhi: Typhim Vi, an injectable polysaccharide vaccine, and Ty21a (Vivotif), an oral live attenuated vaccine. The inactive parenteral vaccine is recommended for PLWH, as the oral typhoid vaccine is a live vaccine that could theoretically cause disseminated disease. Lower immune responses in PLWH to the inactivated vaccine have been reported and correlate with low CD4 counts; efficacy among PLWH is unknown.

POLIO

A single lifetime inactivated polio vaccine booster is recommended among adults at risk for exposure in areas where wild-type virus has not been eradicated in parts of sub-Saharan Africa and Asia. Additional vaccination may be required depending on country-specific requirements; for example, long-term travelers staying within Afghanistan, Nigeria, and Pakistan should receive the polio vaccine between 4 weeks and 12 months before *departure* from these areas where wild-type polio transmission still occurs.

MENINGOCOCCAL DISEASE

Meningococcal vaccination is recommended for all PLWH. Major epidemics of serogroups C and W occur in the "meningitis belt" of Africa. Quadrivalent ACWY vaccine is recommended for travel in areas of transmission during the dry season, December to June. Proof of vaccination is required within the previous 5 years to obtain visas for travel to Saudi Arabia during pilgrimages for Hajj and Umrah.

MEASLES, MUMPS, AND RUBELLA

For adults with newly diagnosed HIV who are without acceptable evidence of MMR immunity, 2 doses of MMR vaccine, given at least 28 days apart, are recommended unless the individuals have evidence of severe immunosuppression (i.e., CD4 percentage < 15% or, if older than 5 years of age, a CD4 count < 200). Acceptable evidence of immunity includes birth before 1957, history of prior vaccination, or laboratory evidence of immunity or disease. Risk for measles transmission is increased in regions with current outbreaks and areas that reside within an antivaccine community.

Administration of MMR vaccine, a live attenuated vaccine, is not recommended in patients with HIV and severe immunosuppression with a CD4 count less than 200. Additionally, administration of the MMR and varicella combination vaccine is not recommended in PLWH as it has not been studied in this population.

JAPANESE ENCEPHALITIS VIRUS

Japanese encephalitis (JE) is an arboviral-borne infection endemic throughout southeast Asia and the western Pacific, with risk of exposure highest in rural agricultural areas. An inactivated vaccine (JE-VC; IXIARO) is available in the United States that protects against all 5 JE virus genotypes. Vaccination is indicated for individuals moving to a JE-endemic country to take up residence, longer term travelers (e.g., ≥ 1 month) to JE-endemic areas, and frequent travelers to JE-endemic areas. The immunogenicity of Japanese encephalitis virus (JEV) vaccination among adults living with HIV is unknown; however, in children living with HIV, most develop seroprotective titers despite reduced antibody responses.

RABIES

Rabies is a virus that can be transmitted to humans by the bite or scratch of a rabid animal (most commonly dogs and bats, but also from a wide range of terrestrial wildlife), resulting in encephalomyelitis that is typically fatal. Rabies is present on every continent except Antarctica, and public health guidance should be sought regarding the risk of rabies after potential exposure by geographic area and animal type. A preexposure rabies vaccine series is recommended for longer stay duration where the rabies threat is heightened in endemic areas of Asia and Africa with limited access to adequate postexposure rabies immunoglobulin and vaccine and for short-term travelers to these areas who engage in adventure activities such as biking, hiking, spelunking, and outdoor running. In case of a high-risk exposure, preexposure vaccination does not eliminate postexposure vaccination, but it simplifies the postexposure vaccine series to two injections, and immunoglobulin is not required.

People living with HIV appear to be at similar risk for rabies, with no known differences in the disease manifestations than HIV-uninfected individuals. US guidelines recommend vaccination among PLWH using the same criteria as for HIV-uninfected persons; a preexposure vaccination series of 3 doses is recommended for those at risk of exposure, with postvaccination serologic testing at 6 months for those at continuous risk and 2 years for those at frequent risk, with a booster dose if antibody titer is below the acceptable level. For postexposure prophylaxis among those without preexposure vaccination, the recommendation is a 5-dose vaccine series at 0, 3, 7, 14, and 28 days (the fifth dose is added for PLWH and other immunocompromised persons vs. the 4-dose series for immunocompetent persons) and human rabies immunoglobulin. Immunogenicity may be reduced among PLWH, especially among those with low CD4 counts, high HIV viral loads, and off ART. In 1 study, 88% of those with a CD4 count greater than 450 on ART developed a protective response after 3 doses of the vaccine. Since responses may vary and persons with even high CD4 counts greater than 500 may not develop protective responses, postvaccination serology should be considered.

CHOLERA

Epidemics of cholera have occurred around the globe, although transmission to travelers is not common. In 2016, Vaxchora (a live attenuated oral cholera vaccine) was approved by the Food and Drug Administration for prevention of cholera caused by serogroup O1 in adults 18 to 64 years of age traveling to affected areas; however, the safety and effectiveness has not been established in immunocompromised individuals. A study of the previously available similar cholera vaccine formulation among PLWH in Mali found that vibriocidal seroconversion was slightly lower among PLWH than HIV-negative participants (58% vs. 71%), with no difference in adverse events. The duration of protection with vaccination beyond 3–6 months is currently unknown for PLWH. No significant differences in occurrence of any systemic adverse events were found between vaccinated and comparison populations. Groups that should be considered for vaccination include aid, refugee, and healthcare workers in endemic and epidemic areas in proximity to displaced populations, especially in crowded camps and urban slums, and if PLWH are involved with such activities and have achieved immune reconstitution with CD4 greater than 200 on effective ART, then vaccination can be considered.

TICK-BORNE ENCEPHALITIS

Tick-borne encephalitis, or TBE, is a human viral infectious disease involving the central nervous system. TBE is caused by the tick-borne encephalitis *Flavivirus*, composed of 3 virus subtypes that indicate their geographic range of activity: European or Western tick-borne encephalitis virus, Siberian tick-borne encephalitis virus, and Far Eastern tick-borne encephalitis virus (formerly known as Russian Spring Summer encephalitis virus), with recent cases also described in the United Kingdom. An additional distinctly evolutionary divergent subtype, Himalayan, has also been described in China since 2018. In endemic areas, recreational or occupational exposure to rural, forested, or outdoor settings among, for example, hunters, campers, forest workers, or farmers during April to October represent risk factors for infection through potential contact with the infected ticks. It is unknown if HIV infection increases the risk for either infection or disease severity. There are data to suggest that deletion in the chemokine receptor 5 (CCR5) gene (i.e., being homozygous for CCR5-Delta 32) is associated with increased risk and severity of flavivirus infections, though whether the use of the CCR5-entry blocker, maraviroc, also increases the risk is unclear. The vaccine is available in most endemic countries, but not in the United States or Canada. The vaccine series is typically with 3 doses; however, British guidelines recommend a 4-dose series (0, 1, 2, and 9–12 months) for PLWH given concerns for possible lower vaccine response rates. Regarding immunogenicity, PLWH, particularly with CD4 counts less than 400, have poorer seroprotective responses compared with HIV-uninfected persons, with vaccine durability unknown. Because the routine primary vaccination series requires 6 months or more for completion, the more practical approach for most travelers going to TBE-endemic areas is avoidance of tick bites than vaccination. For travelers considering vaccination in Europe or Russia on arrival at the destination, a rapid vaccination schedule at 0 and 2 weeks (with a booster dose at 5–12 months) has been evaluated for the European vaccines; however, seroprotective immunity still takes 3 to 4 weeks to develop, making vaccination on arrival impractical for short-stay travelers. There are no data on accelerated vaccination in PLWH. Travelers anticipating high-risk exposures in TBE-endemic countries for extended periods may consider in-country vaccination.

TRAVELER'S DIARRHEA

Diarrheal illness accounts for 20% to 40%, with some estimates up to 70% depending on destination, of reported disease in travelers. Risk is greatest during the first 2 weeks of travel and slowly declines thereafter. Traveler's diarrhea may be caused by various food-borne and waterborne pathogens, the most common include *Salmonella, Campylobacter, Giardia,* and *Cryptosporidium* species and can result in severe illness in immuno-compromised PLWH. Enteroaggregative *Escherichia coli* is an emerging enteric pathogen worldwide that can also cause persistent diarrhea in PLWH. Antibiotic prophylaxis can lead to adverse effects, promote drug resistance, and may contribute to poor judgment among travelers cavalier with their food choices; therefore, it is not recommended, and nonantibiotic prophylaxis requires frequent dosing to achieve only a modest reduction in risk.

Counseling travelers about precautions, such as avoiding food from street stands, tap water, raw foods, and ice does not appear to eliminate the risk of traveler's diarrhea, though washing reduces risk by 30% and alcohol-based hand sanitizer also significantly reduces risk. Overall, a meta-analysis of randomized trials assessing modifying behaviors to preclude contracting diarrheal illness determined there was minimal preventive impact. However, because antibiotics against bacterium that account for most traveler's diarrhea reduce the duration and severity of symptoms (loose stools, cramping, and nausea) and generally are well tolerated, a small carry-along supply for empiric self-treatment can effectively reduce morbidity from diarrheal illness.

Travel destination largely determines antibiotic selection based on patterns of invasive pathogen endemicity and antibiotic resistance surveillance profiles. Although blood in the stool suggests invasive disease, fever is not a sensitive indicator of dysentery. Ciprofloxacin (500 mg twice daily for 1–3 days or an alternative fluoroquinolone) is appropriate for diarrhea contracted in Southeast Asia and Africa due to excellent efficacy against most enteropathogens. Because *Campylobacter* infection is common in Thailand and fluoroquinolone resistance has been reported in 70% to 90% of cases, azithromycin is the treatment of choice. With high resistance rates to SMX-TMP worldwide, it is rarely useful for diarrheal illness outside of that contracted in Mexico or Central America. Rifaximin is an effective drug for noninvasive diarrhea caused by *E. coli*, the predominant pathogen found in Mexico and Central America. There are few concerns over interaction of antibiotic treatment with antiretroviral drugs. Fluoroquinolones have no clinically significant interactions with ART, and azithromycin appears to pose little risk of drug interactions with ART. There are no data available on potential interactions between rifaximin and ART; regardless, rifaximin is a gut luminal agent, with little systemic exposure.

For mild diarrhea, nonantibiotic therapy with loperamide, an antimotility agent, or bismuth subsalicylate, with antisecretory, anti-inflammatory, and antibacterial properties, will usually reduce the number of stools and duration of illness by 50%. For abrupt onset of diarrhea rated beyond mild, in other words causing distress or forcing a change in activities or itinerary, antibiotic therapy can be initiated. If symptoms resolve within 24 hours, no further treatment is necessary. If diarrhea persists after 1 day, treatment should be continued for 1 or 2 more days. Therapy with an antibiotic plus loperamide often limits symptoms to 1 day. Concerns that use of loperamide in dysentery may prolong illness have been outweighed by newer data that now find loperamide safe when combined with an antibiotic. A reasonable strategy for combined loperamide and antibiotic therapy in dysentery is to reserve loperamide for long trips or when the traveler will have no toilet access. For dysentery that fails to respond to 3-day fluoroquinolone or rifaximin therapy, a 3-day course of azithromycin should be introduced. If diarrheal illness persists after azithromycin therapy, stool collection for culture, ova and parasite, and clostridial difficile examination should be obtained, and the traveler should seek medical attention. In general, traveler's diarrhea is not dehydrating, except for the very young, adults aged 65 years or older, or those with chronic medical conditions; nonetheless, all travelers with diarrhea should be encouraged to drink plenty of fluids and to replace lost electrolytes with foods such as salted crackers or broth.

BACK TO THE CASE

After reviewing CDC travel information (https://wwwnc.cdc.gov/travel) for updated travel notices and vaccination requirements, you determine that WT will require YF vaccination for both country entry and protection during hiking activity within an endemic zone. Together with emerging data to treat long-term nonprogressors and elite controllers with ART, and acknowledging that immune responses to YF vaccine are higher with virologic suppression, you encourage WT to start ART. WT agrees and would like the smallest possible pill since he travels extensively and may need to conceal his ART.

With 6 weeks until his trips begins, you feel confident that virologic suppression can be achieved within 2 to 4 weeks given his low baseline viral load after initiating the single-tablet regimen tenofovir alafenamide/emtricitabine/rilpivirine, and then the YF vaccine can be administered at an authorized center between 10 and 14 days before departure. You reassure him that his CD4 is greater than 500 and he is less than 60 years of age to allay safety concerns with the live attenuated vaccine. He is up to date on his routine respiratory (influenza, pneumococcal, and Tdap [tetanus, diphtheria, pertussis) vaccinations and meningococcal disease immunization for PLWH, has documented immunity to hepatitis A, and his isolated positive hepatitis B core antibody indicates past exposure; regardless, the tenofovir and emtricitabine antiretrovirals double as hepatitis B prophylaxis.

You convince him to receive the 3-dose series for rabies preexposure vaccination as his itinerary includes hiking in remote Ugandan mountains and plan to check a 6-month postvaccination titer since his business is going well, and he will likely venture into similar excursions in the future. You discuss overall mosquito bite prevention, including permethrin-embedded bed nets and use of DEET repellent. WT prefers atovaquone/proguanil malaria prophylaxis with fewer comparative side effects, and there are no drug-drug interactions with his new ART. For only a 2-week trip, you do not encourage additional SMX-TMP prophylaxis. You provide him a 3-day supply of ciprofloxacin, and along with reviewing safe eating and drinking precautions, you explain the algorithm for antibiotic use in case of a diarrheal illness. Bon voyage!

KEY POINTS TO REMEMBER

- Traveler's diarrhea is the most common infection among international travelers; antibiotic prophylaxis is not recommended, but short -course empiric self-treatment with a fluoroquinolone, rifaximin, or azithromycin (depending on the destination region) for moderate-to-severe diarrheal illness can reduce morbidity.
- Live attenuated vaccines should be avoided in PLWH if an inactivated form of the vaccine is available. However, asymptomatic PLWH with CD4 greater than 200 have limited immune deficits for vaccination purposes, so administration of live attenuated vaccination for PLWH who cannot avoid travel to areas with risk for infection can be considered generally safe.
- All travelers are at risk for respiratory illnesses from person-to-person transmission, and pretravel health consultation is an opportunity to ensure all routine vaccinations for PLWH are up to date.
- Extra precautions are needed for PLWH planning travel to countries with entry restrictions to protect against disclosure and potential interruptions of ART.

Further Reading

Barte H, Horvath TH, Rutherford GW. Yellow fever vaccine for patients with HIV infection. *Cochrane Database Syst Rev.* 2014;(1):CD010929. doi:10.1002/14651858. CD010929.pub2

Campbell JD, Moore D, Degerman R, et al. HIV-infected Ugandan adults taking antiretroviral therapy with CD4 counts > 200 cells/μL who discontinue cotrimoxazole prophylaxis have increased risk of malaria and diarrhea. *Clin Infect Dis.* 2012;54(8):1204–1211.

Centers for Disease Control and Prevention. Travelers' health. https://wwwnc.cdc.gov/travel

Crum-Cianflone NF, Sullivan E. Vaccinations for the HIV-infected adult. A review of the current recommendations, part II. *Infect Dis Ther.* 2017;6:333–361.

DuPont HL, Mattila L. Antimicrobial treatment: an algorithmic approach. In: Ericsson CD, DuPont HL, Steffen R, eds. *Travelers' Diarrhea.* Hamilton, Canada: Decker; 2003:227–237.

Freeman DO, Chen LH. Vaccines for international travel. *Mayo Clin Proc.* 2019;94(11):2314–2339.

The Global Database on HIV-Specific Travel and Residence Restrictions. Home page. https://www.hivtravel.org

UNAIDS. UNAIDS and UNDP call on 48* countries and territories to remove all HIV-related travel restrictions. https://www.unaids.org/en/resources/presscentre/press releaseandstatementarchive/2019/june/20190627_hiv-related-travel-restrictions

World Health Organization. International travel and health: information about yellow fever vaccination requirement. https://www.who.int/ith/ith_country_list.pdf

Index